Inflammation & Diet: Healing Arthritis with Food

1# ARTHRITIS: Understanding Arthritis, Its Prevention & Reversal With A Sirt Food & Plant Based Diet

2# SIRT FOOD: The Secret Behind Nutrition, Healthy Weight Loss, Disease Prevention, Reversal & Longevity

By John Hodges & Ted Gif

www.viddapublishing.com

This edition published by
VIDDA Publishing Ltd in 2016. www.viddapublishing.com
Copyright © VIDDA Publishing Ltd 2016

Cover design by John Hodges.

VIDDA Publishing BOOK SHELF:
www.viddapublishing.com/books.html

Your FREE Gift

Thank you for purchasing this book. To show our appreciation we would like to offer you a FREE copy of our eBook: "**A Complete Handbook of NATURE CURES**".

To download, go to **viddapublishing_0.gr8.com/**

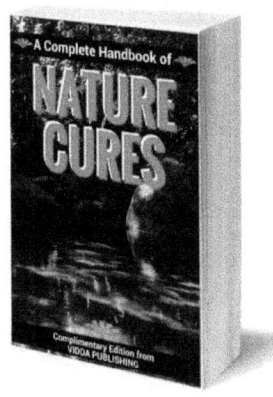

If you're interested in Health, Nutrition, Green and / or Cruelty Free products please visit our Websites and online **VIDDA Health Stores** (US: bit.ly/VIDDAstore & UK: bit.ly/VIDDAstoreUK).

www.viddapublishing.com

www.sirtfood.com

www.themedicineonyourplate.com

www.greenupyourlife.org

www.ecologizatuvida.com

Table of Content

ARTHRITIS: Understanding Arthritis, Its Prevention & Reversal With A Sirt Food & Plant Based Diet

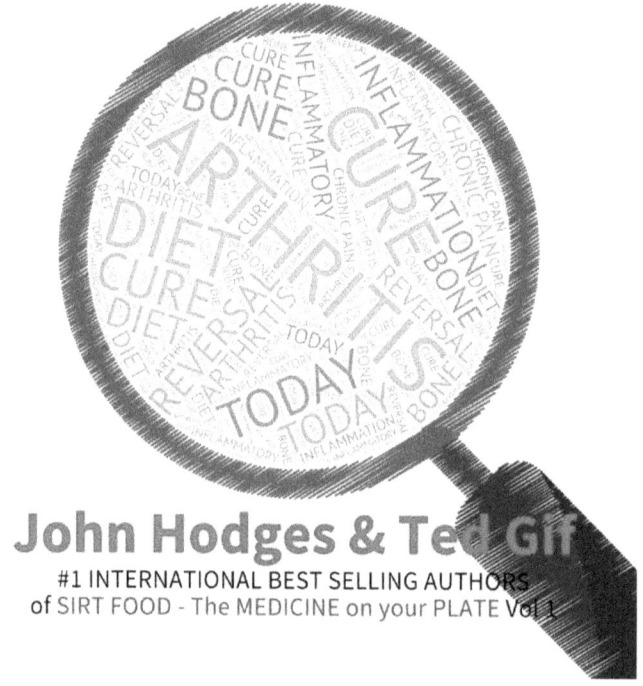

The MEDICINE on your Plate - vol 4

ARTHRITIS

Understanding Arthritis,
its Prevention & Reversal
with a SIRT FOOD & Plant Based Diet

John Hodges & Ted Gif

#1 INTERNATIONAL BEST SELLING AUTHORS
of SIRT FOOD - The MEDICINE on your PLATE Vol 1

Introduction

Arthritis has hundreds of forms and therefore possible causes but for our purposes we will be focusing on the two most common forms which are Osteoarthritis (OA) and Rheumatoid Arthritis (RA). To fully appreciate the negative impact of arthritis it is crucial that the reader gain an overview of the workings of the systems of the human body that the disease affects. Such systems and the processes which ensure they function properly will be discussed throughout the text, but much of this knowledge will be imparted in chapter one. In essence to really understand the wholly negative impacts of arthritis an understanding of the formation and function materials such as bone and cartilage is crucial.

Chapter two and three will discuss the differences between the two forms of arthritis which in general terms are analogous to the differences between Type-1 and Type-2 diabetes discussed in the "diabetes" book. Hence for reasons that will become clear chapter two will begin with an outline of how the immune system works and what is meant by an "autoimmune disease", this latter term was defined in "diabetes", here it will be outlined in some detail.

Chapter four will focus on the degree to which being overweight or obese influences the onset of both forms of arthritis. Clearly, the term obesity is an emotive and complex subject and has been discussed to varying degrees in all texts presented in these volumes. The reader is encouraged to see the condition as a key driver for many negative health conditions. I will impart again that in our context we are not discussing obesity that is due to side effects from medical treatment or a mental health issue. We are talking solely about obesity that is preventable on daily basis by the individual concerned changing their lifestyle and dietary choices.

Finally chapter five will discuss some of the active compounds, nutrients, mineral substances and food groups which are believed to have a role in "*arthritis*". The food groups indicated do not constitute an exhaustive list and so the reader is encouraged to carry out their own research, using the references and hyperlinks as a starting point. This final chapter will explain the role of positive diet and lifestyle choices in the prevention of arthritis. Overall, the reader will appreciate the difference between both forms of arthritis. In addition, wherever I have felt it necessary to do so I have differentiated between both forms of the disease, well at least the two forms that are under discussion here. Overall, wherever you read the word "arthritis" you can assume that we are talking about both conditions interchangeably. The message running though all of these books is that there is nothing inevitable about a whole host of health conditions and that by adopting the contained advice you can reduce your risk of developing such a condition and arthritis is no different. So let's get to it, shall we?

Chapter 1:
Introducing the Skeletal System

The word arthritis is derived from a fusion of Latin and Greek and literally means a disease of the joints, tissues and fluids which enable them (the joints) to function properly. At the earliest possible juncture I have decided to make as absolutely clear as the azure blue sky on the sunniest day you can imagine, that there is no cure for the disease. Arthritis is a progressive, debilitating and degenerative disease that causes harm to the people that have the misfortune to develop it. Arthritis is not as life threatening as a disease such as cancer but if left unchecked the condition will severely degrade the quality of life of sufferers and those around them. Arthritis is one of the most common joint diseases in the world but is more common in the northern and Caucasian countries. However, the incidence of the disease is rising in all countries with an ageing population.

According to the UK National Health Service (NHS) the condition affects approximately 10 million people in the UK alone. There are several UK based charities which support, campaign, research, and otherwise promote the condition as a major negative impact on public health. The two most common forms of the disease are osteoarthritis (OA) and Rheumatoid Arthritis (RA) and will be discussed in chapters two and three respectively. At this juncture it is sufficient to impart that the OA is more prevalent than RA by a factor of about 10, at least in the UK. In 2009 According to a UK charity (www.Arthritisresearchuk.org) some 9 million people sought treatment for OA. Almost all the remaining one million sufferers sought help for RA. It is important to realise that these conditions are but two of the 150-200 separate conditions which fall into the category of Rheumatic or musculoskeletal disease. Such estimates around the world are difficult to quantify but the total is certainly in the few hundred million. In the US approximately 50 million people are believed experience arthritis which includes about 300,000 children, that is people under 18 years old. Interestingly, in the US "only" about twice as many people suffer with OA as opposed to RA. Overall, arthritis progresses from a position of enforced limited movement and locomotion to the extreme of needing constant support, where the person loses their independence.

As animals and plants increase in size and complexity the need for a support, movement and locomotion system becomes ever more apparent. In biology a structure which enables these three requirements is known as a skeleton. The skeleton provides all animals (including ourselves) with the distinctive shape by which all vertebrate organisms are recognised. Organisms such as human beings with an internal skeletal structure are said to have an endo-skeleton. The type of skeleton an organism has is used to help taxonomists classify the biosphere, for example any invertebrate organism with an exo-skeleton belongs to the phylum (division) called the arthropods. Overall in vertebrate organisms the musculoskeletal system works together as a system of levers. The bones, muscles ligaments and tendons allow the animal to push against its external environment (i.e. the ground, air or water). Thus we all prove Isaac Newton's third law of motion as we travel along with our bipedalism that is we walk on two legs! If you have a domesticated animal for a pet it is likely to travel in a quadrupedal fashion i.e. Fido and / or Felix walk on four legs. Walking and movement occurs because every time a force is applied an equal but opposite force works in the opposite direction. In other words we are able to undergo locomotion (movement of the whole organism) due to the resistance produced when we push against our external environment. This of course is why space walking, despite the danger, looks so much fun.

The skeleton holds the human organism together, enabling its organ systems to function as they should and allows the muscles to contract, thus carrying out movement. As we maintain our shape we are subject to mechanical forces which generate different stresses on the body. It goes without saying that most organisms are subject to similar stresses, for example:

- It is easier to support a large organism in a marine or aquatic environment than on the land, water is relatively speaking a much more supportive medium.

- Organisms need to resist the impact of physical environmental forces such as wind air pressure, waves and currents.

- As we move (undergo locomotion) we alter the above said forces and so the organism must be adapted to cope with this.

In terms of physics stress takes three broad forms. First compression is a function of objects pushing against each other, tension occurs when they pull apart from each other and shear occurs when objects try to slide over each other. All organisms have evolved and adapted to incorporate these changes and so the physical and biological worlds are inextricably linked.

As well as support the skeleton also has a protective function. For instance, the brain is protected from impact injury by the skull whilst the heart is protected by the sternum and lungs by the rib cage. The spinal cord is protected by a structure known as the neural arch, which is specific adaptation running through the back bone. The bones allow movement and locomotion by acting as biological levers such that when the muscles pull (they never push) on bones and movement is the result, hence the term muscular locomotion. Such processes enable the intercostal muscles to pull on the ribs whilst we inspire and expire air from the lungs i.e. undergo breathing and the masseter muscles enable us to chew our food. For the skeletal muscles to produce such movement, both ends of a given muscle must be attached to the bone. The skeleton has evolved to provide points of attachment for the skeletal muscles. Put simply, ligaments attach bones to other bones and tendons attach muscle to bones. As was outlined in the *"SIRT FOOD"* and *"cancer"* books, the skeleton is a site for the production of red blood and white blood cells. In between the supporting matrix of spongy bone are the hemocytoblasts which become the red and white blood cells. We recognise this structure as the bone marrow and the principle sites of red blood cell production are the heads of the limbs, the ribs and the vertebrae. Due to the detrimental effects on the skeleton, both OA and RA can have a negative impact on any number of these functions. Which to put it succinctly is why arthritis is such an undesirable biological development.

In biology the back bone or vertebral column supports the skull (cranium) which contains the brain. The human vertebral column is an arrangement of 33 individual vertebra (plural vertebrae) which are separated by discs of a fibrous tissue we know as cartilage, allowing the vertebral column a degree of flexibility. Cartilage which covers the surface of bones is soft, smooth and slippery but is also very cohesive and firm. A *"slipped disc"* occurs when the vertebra are able to press directly against the spinal cord. Such an occurrence is as painful as it is undesirable and is generally one of the physical signs of ageing. In short as we get older the discs of cartilage start to lose water and harden as they do so, the process makes them progressively less flexible and more likely to move and / or rupture.

Under normal circumstances cartilage is not hardened by the deposition of calcium phosphate Ca_3 $(PO_4)_2$ crystals, the principal compound which gives bone its hardness. Joints are the points of the skeletal system where our bones join together. Hyaline cartilage is the most common type and it covers the surface area of the bones which form the major joints in the body. At these junctures the cartilage works as a natural shock absorber and also enables the bones to slide over each other, without them being damaged by friction. Hyaline cartilage is in essence a very tightly woven matrix of collagen fibres which in living organisms has a slight blue tint. In ossification (bone formation) and skeletal development it is hyaline cartilage that is converted to bone. Hyaline cartilage serves the body by joining bones such as the ribs and Sternum (amongst others) to each other. Structurally, elastic cartilage is identical to hyaline cartilage, it just serves different functions. For example the epiglottis, ear lobes and tip and bridge of nose are all made of elastic cartilage. In broad terms we can say that Elastic cartilage has a connective and supportive role, whilst hyaline cartilage has a lubricating and absorbing role. You can appreciate the properties of cartilage by squashing the tip of your nose or pulling on your ear lobes. The importance of cartilage can further be acknowledged by asking yourself *"how can I swallow without the epiglottis or breathe without a trachea and effective bronchial network?"* A third form of cartilage known as fibrocartilage is the most densely wrapped matrix of all and is found where extra durability is required.

The cushioning of knee joint are two biological structures cushioned by fibrocartilage.

Cartilage itself is derived from a class of cells known as the chondrocytes which secrete a jelly substance which surrounds and then encapsulates them. The more chondrocytes the cartilage contains the more flexible it is. Cartilage is unique among the connective tissues because it is not supplied by the capillaries of the circulatory system. In other words the chondrocytes are segregated from each other and from a direct nutrition supply, as provided by the circulatory system. Furthermore, if cartilage is damaged it takes longer to heal because the appropriate substances must travel through the bones themselves. The chondrocytes are situated in miniscule cavities called the lacuna and so when damage occurs or any form of nutrient exchange is needed substances must move by diffusion (which requires liquid) from the immediate environment surrounding the chondrocyte to the blood plasma and back again. Such a movement is much slower than having direct contact with the blood as happens during a cut or contusion to the skin. This reality presents a further complication in both the prevention and treatment of arthritis.

For all mammals the development of a functioning skeleton is absolutely essential for the success of the organism. Hence it is not surprising that in human beings bone formation starts during the gestation of the foetus and continues until the end of adolescence, when the skeleton stops growing. This is not the same as the process of bone resorption and remodelling which continues throughout the life of the person. In essence the working of the skeleton is a function of two complex processes resorption and ossification. Resorption is the breakdown of worn, damaged or older bone and is unique to the osteoclast cells discussed below. At any given time in a healthy adult skeleton about 10% of the bone tissue is undergoing resorption. Ossification is the formation of new bone and is absolutely key to maintaining the shape of the skeleton and to the repair of injury (fractures and breakage). There are three types of bone cell.

The osteoblasts are the cells found on the surface of the bone and are responsible for bone formation. They produce a substance called osteoid, which is almost entirely collagen and are located inside the lacunae (plural of lacuna). These specialist cells secrete an enzyme called alkaline phosphatase which facilitates the deposition of calcium (Ca^{2+}) and phosphate (PO_4^-) ions. When these ions combine to form crystals of $Ca_3(PO_4)_2$ the osteoid becomes mineralised and the result is bone. A mineral is defined as any naturally occurring compound with a well-defined crystal structure. Mineralisation refers to a process whereby a living organism produces an inorganic (mineral) substance, in the case of bone formation the substance is $Ca_3(PO_4)_2$. In bone mineralisation this compound is integrated into the collagen matrix and the whole process is regulated by a substance called inorganic (non-carbon based) pyrophosphate. Bone formation is often called calcification and the pyrophosphate ensures that it occurs as it should, where it should and at the rate it should. Overall then, the osteoid is hardened into what biologists call an ossified matrix, which is composed of water, proteins and salts of calcium and phosphorous. After the bone has completely ossified (hardened) the living cells are able to communicate with each other via miniscule channels called canaliculi.

The osteocytes are essentially the same as the osteoblasts but are located underneath the surface of the bone. They function by ensuring that the correct level (homeostasis) of oxygen and $Ca_3(PO_4)_2$ are maintained during bone formation. The osteoclasts are responsible for the resorption of bone. At specific sites on the surface of the bone the phosphatase acid is secreted by the osteoclasts. The acid breaks the chemical bonds between the calcium and phosphate ions, thus breaking down the $Ca_3 (PO_4)_2$ into its constituent elements. In metabolism if an element is useful to the body it will generally be recycled by the organism as opposed to being excreted. So in this process the calcium, oxygen and phosphate ions are reused. Overall bone is a tough and resilient mixture of proteins and minerals and is the material responsible for the strength of the skeleton. Bone is a hard strong structure designed to resist impact, bending and compression, not bad for a substance which is 20% water!

What is not often realised is that bone is living tissue composed of cells which constantly reproduce. The durable properties of bone are derived from the polymerised crystals of $Ca_3 (PO_4)_2$. The entire skeleton as with all living tissue is permeated by the capillaries of the circulatory system. The capillaries are the tiny blood vessels which support every single cell in the body. In other words nutrients are supplied, waste products of metabolism are removed and the all-important processes of growth and repair take place. The human skeleton is composed of two basic types of bone, as one can infer the outer layer of our bones is composed of a hard, dense structure known as compact or cortical bone. Underneath this layer is a spongy structure referred to as Cancellous or Trabecular bone. This internal structure is interspersed with thousands of struts of cortical bone thus forming a honeycombed network which supports the outer layer. The cortical bone is cylindrical in shape and in effect surrounds the spongy bone and accounts for some 4/5th's of the total mass of the bone, the remaining 20% of bone is made of the spongy bone. The organisation of each different bone is derived from how it is evolved to carry out its particular function. For instance, the thigh bone is subjected to the stresses caused by bending, but the bones of the inner ear are designed to transmit sound waves to the auditory nerves. Hence they have different amounts and distributions of both cortical and trabecular bone. The thickness of the spongy bone varies according to the function of the bone and overall the more tensile and / or compressive stress the bone is subjected to, the more spongy bone is present. The human skeleton is adapted such that the minimum quantity of cortical bone tissue is needed to provide the maximum degree of strength and support.

Bone forms initially from fibres of a protein called collagen which is the principle connective tissue in the human body. Overall collagen is the most common protein to be found in mammals. Collagen is the building material from which all bone is constructed and it comprises about 30% of all the protein to be found in a person. The role of collagen in the body is crucially important to our understanding of arthritis in all in its forms. Each collagen fibre is composed of a chain of about 1000 amino acids (the molecules from which all proteins are made). As we shall see collagen is easily damaged by a number of risk factors including but not limited to, excessive sugar in the diet, tobacco smoke and alcohol. Collagen has a triple helix structure with the individual fibres intertwined about each other. Across the entire structure are specific sites which allow for the formation of the calcium phosphate crystals. Bone also contains carbonates (any compound which contains CO_3^{2-} ions) of zinc and silicon. The bones of younger people have a higher collagen content than those of older people, thus explaining why *"younger"* bone is generally more flexible than *"older"* bone. The bones of a healthy adult skeletal system are approximately 70% $Ca_3(PO_4)_2$ and about 30% collagen. Furthermore, collagen is found in the dermis (inner layers) of the skin and it provides extra elasticity to the nerves, blood vessels and the mucous membranes found throughout the body. Collagen as well as being essential for bone formation has a high tensile strength and so is the perfect material for making tendons and ligaments. Finally, collagen surrounds and protects the softer organs of the body such as the spleen and kidneys. All things considered collagen is more than essential for your good health. The negative impacts of arthritis as a whole are collectively some of the principle reasons why the disease is so detrimental to human health.

The types of muscle which are important for our context are voluntary (skeletal) muscle and involuntary muscle. The cardiac muscles of the heart and coronary arteries will not be discussed in this book. The voluntary muscle is composed of long individual muscle fibres which have fused together. Under a microscope the cell membrane and nucleus are present but only the latter cellular structure is visible. The fibres themselves are best seen as bundles connected to the nervous system such that when the muscle receives an electrical impulse (nervous signal) the muscle will contract becoming more compact and wider than in the relaxed state. Under most circumstances we can control these muscles, hence the term voluntary muscle. Although they are the same structure, the involuntary muscles tend to form layers as opposed to a definite form of muscle. Examples include the layers which form the walls of the oesophagus, the uterus and the arterioles. All muscles will contract (shorten) when they receive the nervous impulse to do so. Muscles cannot push, they can only pull, hence they cannot elongate further from a fully relaxed position. So for movement or locomotion to occur a muscle is pulled to a compressed position, contributing to the movement, before it is allowed to return to the relaxed (elongated) state.

The ends of the muscles are drawn out into tendons which firmly attach a given muscle to the skeleton. The tendon at one end of a muscle is attached to a part of the skeleton which does not move, whilst at the other the tendon is attached to moveable bone close to but not part of the joint. When the nervous impulse *"tells"* the muscle to pull the bone the skeleton will move. The tendon is attached such that the physical law of moments is applied, in other words the tiny contraction of the muscle produces a large movement at the end of the muscle. The text book example is the relationship between the biceps, the top voluntary muscle in the upper arm and the triceps, the bottom voluntary muscles. If you place your arms out palms up and then bring your fingers to your shoulders the following process unfolds. The contraction of the biceps flexes the arm at the elbow, whilst simultaneously the tricep straightens and extends to its maximum length. If you bring your palms back to their starting position the opposite occurs. The non-moving end of the bicep is attached to the shoulder blade and the moving end is attached to the ulna bone, near the elbow hinge joint. The muscles which make the limbs move are arranged in pairs which move in opposite directions when the impulse to move is sent from the brain. The tricep pulls the compressed bicep back to its original elongated position. Muscles pairs which work in this way are known as antagonistic pairs, when one muscle contracts the other relaxes. In addition to allowing movement and locomotion the process keeps both muscles in an equilibrium tension. Antagonistic pairs do not always cause locomotion, for example chewing, breathing, swallowing and blinking are all examples of movement that do not result in locomotion.

Overall more than one of these processes, structures or systems can be disrupted or even destroyed by the development of either RA or OA. Furthermore, there is no biological reason why any of the 200 rheumatologically debilitating syndromes are mutually exclusive. In other words it is possible to develop more than one condition at the same time. No doubt about it arthritis is not a trivial condition, quite the opposite is true!

Chapter 2:
What is Rheumatoid Arthritis?

RA is an example of an autoimmune disease; it is significantly rarer than OA which is generally associated with the physical symptoms of ageing. RA is a chronic and debilitating disease which can affect the joints in any part of the skeletal system, most commonly the hands, wrists, and knees. According to the British Society of Rheumatology about 700,000 people are experiencing some degree of RA and 20,000 new cases are diagnosed every year. In addition 12,000 cases of juvenile idiopathic arthritis (juvenile RA) are diagnosed on an annual basis. Overall the symptoms begin to express themselves in middle age and about 75% of sufferers are women Thus, indicating a genetic predisposition to the condition which may be linked to the menopause. The condition is far more common in women of the minority world (The US, Europe and Australia). For researchers in the field of rheumatology (study of inflammatory disease) there is strong evidence that many metabolic pathways are implicated in the expression of RA. A perusal of the research literature will impart that ever more individual and classes of biological, cell signalling and even hormonal molecules are involved in the onset of RA. However, no single trigger has yet been established and it is likely that this will never be the case; RA is believed to be too complex a condition for this eventuality. Before any overview of the pathology and possible prevention of RA (and autoimmune disease in general) can be provided, the human immune system must be discussed.

When it is functioning normally the immune system serves the body by eliminating all foreign substances as quickly as it can. In an autoimmune response, this system breaks down such that the immune system attacks specific cells (and tissues or organs of the body). In this frame the prefix "auto" is derived from the Greek word for "self", thus an autoimmune response is a situation whereby the body attacks itself at a molecular and cellular level. Type-1 diabetes, discussed in *"diabetes"*, is an autoimmune disease. Other examples include Multiple Sclerosis (MS), which destroys the insulating layer (myelin sheath) of central nervous system cells. The result is a steady accumulation of scar tissue which progressively degrades the impulse transmitting function of the affected cells. Crohn's disease occurs when the internal absorbing surface of the intestines is destroyed a further example is a glomerulonephritis which rapidly degrades the filtering abilities of the kidneys. The injury which ensues from most autoimmune diseases is often permanent because the affected cells cannot regenerate. It is estimated that hundreds of millions of people around the world are affected by autoimmune diseases. In many ways, they can be just as life-threatening and /or incapacitating as hereditary disease and for most there is no cure. Some autoimmune disease is more prevalent in certain populations than in others. For example, a collective of autoimmune diseases termed lupus is more common in African and Hispanic women (and women overall) than Caucasian women. If you have lupus, the immune system produces antibodies to many different types of cells and so it causes inflammation in many different organs and so damages

21

different organ systems. When any autoimmune response occurs the immune system *"views"* its own antigens (autoantigens) as foreign antigens and some form of tissue or organ damage resulting in harm to the person is the result. An antigen is any chemical substance which causes the body to produce antibodies against it, hence to explain this we must widen the writing to provide an overview of the human immune system. Such a position will also enable you to gain a deeper understanding of the biological consequences of arthritis.

The human immune system functions by protecting the cells of the body against attack by foreign (i.e. non-human) organisms. These organisms can be unicellular, parasites, bacteria or viruses. In turn, they may or may not be pathogenic (harmful) and may (or may not) cause long-term damage to the person. The health of the immune system is directly linked to the health of the circulatory system (including the lymphatic system) and the principal structures involved in its workings are the spleen, thymus gland and various types of white blood and specialist immune cells. An immune response occurs when the cells of the immune system detect the foreign substances attached to or secreted from the non-human organisms; these substances are collectively termed foreign antigens. The equivalent substances produced by your cells are termed autoantigens. The immune system produces antibodies which are designed to attack and destroy the *"foreign agency"*. The antibodies are specific to each individual foreign agency, such that the antibodies which recognise the typhoid bacteria will not recognise the antigens produced by the pneumonia bacteria. The term lymphocyte is applied to any white blood cell which has the ability to *"recognise"* specific antigens. The lymphocytes in effect patrol the lymphatic system and are split into two broad classes:

B-lymphocytes: These are produced in the bone marrow and migrate directly to the lymph nodes. In the presence of a specific antigen, they reproduce rapidly and secrete an excess of the necessary antibodies which will destroy the *"invading"* biological entity. The really clever part is that although these cells only have a lifespan of a few days, the immune system has adapted to leave behind *"memory cells"* in the lymph nodes. Should the same antigens be recognised the immune system responds such that sufficient antibodies are produced before the *"invader"* has any chance to exert its detrimental and / or toxic effects. The memory cells are the biological basis for acquired immunity.

T-lymphocytes: The prefix T refers to the fact that these cells are produced in the bone marrow but are transported to the thymus gland where they mature. A healthy thymus is able to filter out those T cells which would potentially adversely react to its own cells. Once they have matured the T cells migrate from the thymus gland to the lymphatic system or specific organs of the body. There are three types of T cell and all play a pivotal role in the immune system.

I.   Helper Cells: These cells activate white blood cells and also secrete marker chemicals called opsonins which attach themselves to the foreign antigens. Once this occurs the *"invader"* is literally marked for death by phagocytosis.

II.   Killer Cells: These recognise cells which have been invaded by virus particles by disrupting the cell membrane causing the compromised cell to lose its contents. For example by releasing minute quantities of hydrogen peroxide.

III. Suppressor Cells: These cells switch off the immune response to the foreign *"invader"* has been destroyed.

Overall the B and T cells cooperate and in the absence of an autoimmune condition are highly adept at removing *"foreign molecules"* should they enter the body. Clearly, as conditions such as Ebola, HIV and the syndrome it causes show us, the human immune system is not invincible. All B and T lymphocytes travel through the circulatory system which ensures that they are distributed throughout the body. All cells carry antigens and all things being equal, the body can tell the difference between *"you"* and *"alien"* antigens. Aside from identical twins no two people carry exactly the same antigens but once a *"foreigner"* enters the body there is an immediate response from the immune system. In very general terms the B cells first recognise the *"invader"* and expose its antigens and then the helper T cells release cytokines (cell communication molecules) which *"tell"* the B cells to rapidly reproduce and release the antibodies which will destroy the *"invader"*. Their secondary role is to fire up the white blood cells (phagocytes) to *"fight"* more aggressively. Only mature lymphocytes can work in this capacity and the majority are produced before the end of puberty. In addition, because each cell is designed to fight one infection, the human immune system is able to rapidly respond to millions of different pathogens.

As a human foetus gestates and we grow and mature to the end of adolescence the immune system develops such that the lymphocytes which could attack autoantigens are deleted. This state of affairs is maintained unless autoantigens are mutated and / or specific cells or tissues are altered by the foreign antigens. If tissue-specific autoantigens do not develop then it is likely that the lymphocytes will *"confuse"* those particular cells and see them as *"foreign"* and an autoimmune disease is a result. When tissues and organs become damaged the first response is inflammation and the response is triggered by the cells themselves, which release a class of chemicals called histamines. It is anti-histamines that suppress the allergic response to asthma or hay fever. In asthma the immune response causes the breathing difficulties, unsurprisingly its scientific term is *"acute inflammatory response"*. It is brought about by the narrowing of the airways and the rush of white blood cells to the bronchi.

As of 2015, the full nature of autoimmune diseases has yet to be understood, however, there is very strong evidence that infection by pathogens plays a major role if an individual has a genetic disposition toward such an eventuality. It is this scenario which is widely considered to occur with type-1 diabetes and RA. Other possible mechanisms include *"molecular mimicry"*. As the term suggests a foreign molecule can bear such a close similarity to a specific autoantigen that antibodies are still produced because the *"invader"* is recognised as such. However, the cells of the body which resemble the body have auto-antigens which are so similar that they, in turn, are also destroyed. Another similar mechanism is a fusion of the foreign and autoantigens which in turns activates an immune response. If the inflammatory molecules are present when a lymphocyte is presented with an autoantigen by a foreign molecule, then the lymphocytes can be *"tricked"* into attacking the specific cells. Any somatic cells in possession of that antigen are then destroyed. OK, thanks for paying attention to the biology, now we can go back to arthritis!

RA occurs when the immune system targets the bones, connective tissue (ligaments and tendons) and cartilage of the joints causing inflammation, pain, and deformity of the skeletal shape. In other words, both of these essential tissues and the specialist cells they are composed of are seen as *"foreign"* and attacked by the immune system. The B and T cells of the immune system travel throughout the body by virtue of the circulatory system and so RA can express itself on the site of any single joint on the skeletal system. The pain and discomfort caused by RA are a direct consequence of the inflammatory response which we feel as stiffness, swelling, pain, heat and varying degrees of pain within the affected joints. If you are experiencing these sensations for more than an hour then a visit to your GP, doctor or physician is required! A genetic association for RA was first put forward in 1987 where peptides (a molecule made of two or more amino acids chemically bonded to each other) with a specific orientation and electrical charge were shown to interact with T cells, initiating the autoimmune response.

Further research has revealed that molecules called citrullinated proteins are the subject of attack by anti-cyclic citrullinated protein antibodies. These antibodies are well recognised by scientists being specific for the autoimmune response which expresses itself as RA. A further indicator is the presence of a biological marker called the HLA shared epitope. The epitope is that part of an antigen where the antibody attaches itself. The acronym HLA means *"human leukocyte antigen"* which is that part of the human genome which codes for the proteins involved in the human immune system. Overall this particular molecule has been directly associated with a fivefold increase in the risk of developing RA, as compared to people without it. Other genes are also known to increase the risk but it is important to state that even if such genes are present, the person will not (all variables considered) definitely develop RA. The reason is simple, no causative link for RA has been established and so here we are concerned with the assessment of risk and the influence of environmental, hormonal and dietary factors.

In the "cancer," book mention was made of cells known as macrophages in the development of breast cancer. The same is true of RA; in short, the first stage of RA is penetration of the synovial membrane (the synovium) by the macrophages. Once inside the synovial fluid the macrophages activate biochemical called major histocompatibility complex (MHC) molecules and secrete a wide range of other chemicals which promote inflammation. From here a whole series of biochemical reactions occurs which require a Ph.D. in the subject to fully understand. Suffice to say the activity of the macrophages disrupts the normal activity of the synovial fluid. Afterwards, RA progresses to the joint itself whereby B cells begin to attack the chondrocytes and osteoblasts. Needless to say, the swelling and pain intensifies and joint functionality degrades as the disease spreads. RA is a condition which has a particular affinity for the synovial (movable) joints such as the elbow, knee, wrists, fingers and vertebrae. The negative impacts range from pain and discomfort to a situation where pressure on the spine can induce symptoms akin to paralysis and as such can be life threatening. Overall the end point of RA is a total disintegration of the joint and the supporting structures. Hence movement impossible terrible agony and contortion occurs, make no mistake late stage RA is a nasty and unpleasant condition. RA can also cause swelling of the lymph nodes and cause negative impacts on other organs (the skin, eyes, lungs and heart) and other systems of the human body.

Aside from genetic factors, the chemicals found in cigarette smoke have been implicated in the onset of RA for decades. The chemicals contained in cigarette smoke are known to accelerate the hardening of cartilage. In particular carbon monoxide, the hydrocarbons (which are identical to those produced in combustion engines) and nicotine itself are thought to promote an autoimmune response by tricking the immune system into attacking the citrullinated proteins found in the joints. Put simply, even if you are following the best anti-inflammatory diet in the world, the more you smoke the greater is the risk of developing RA, especially if you are female and menopausal. So, sticking with the good cheer let us move on to chapter four.

Chapter 3:
What is Osteoarthritis?

The human skeleton is made of 206 bones held together by a system of joints, of which there are three basic types. In no particular order, an example of a fixed (immovable) joint system are the sutural joints of the cranium. Movable or synovial joints are the primary targets of RA. Hence the joints of the elbow, where the humerus (upper arm bone), ulna and radius (lower arm bones) meet or the knee, where the femur (thigh) and tibia (shin) bones meet are two examples of vulnerable joints. Other examples of these hinge joints include those which enable the fingers to flex and move and the wrist to turn, allowing the movement of the hands to *"palm up"* or *"palm down"* positions. Each of our femur bones is attached to the pelvis by a ball and socket joint whilst at the knee, it forms another hinge joint via the tibia. Ball and socket joints such as those at the junctions of the hip and shoulders, which allow forward, backward and sideways movement, are vulnerable to both principle forms of arthritis. Where they meet all bones are held in place by ligaments which hold the bones in place but do not contribute to their movement. The ligaments are composed of collagen and another protein-based connective tissue called elastin. OA is a serious and wholly undesirable condition which progressively destroys the joints by destroying the cartilage which enables them to function properly. Furthermore, cartilage is avascular (not connected to the circulatory system) making the disease even more difficult to treat.

Taken together the skull and spinal column are sometimes referred to as an axial skeleton and the limb girdles and bones are termed as the appendicular skeleton. From the vertebral column, twelve pairs of ribs encase and protect the lungs. The two pairs of limbs are attached to the spine by virtue of structures called girdles. The Pelvic girdle joins the lower point of the spine to the bones of the legs. The shoulder (pectoral) girdle is composed of a pair of collarbones and shoulder blades. These are not attached directly to the spine but are held in place by muscles. The humerus fits into a socket space inside the shoulder blade, similarly, the femur fits into a larger socket inside the pelvis. The cranium protects and encases the brain and carries the primary sense organs, (the eyes, ears, nose, and mouth). The base of the skull forms a joint system (the atlas and axis) with the top of the vertebrae which allows the head to move. We are then able to communicate non-verbally and gain an aural and visual awareness of our surroundings. The upper jaw (a fixed joint) is attached to the skull but the lower jaw moves by virtue of a specifically evolved hinge joint. This particular adaption allows us to chew the food we ingest and facilitates the first stages of digestion. Any of these joints can be affected by the onset of OA. The synovial joints possess a thin layer of a thick, viscous liquid substance, (laden with specialist proteins) known as a synovial fluid which further reduces friction by increasing the degree of lubrication. Think of the way hydraulic pistons work in vehicles and their need for specialist synthetic oils and you should get the idea! The fluid also contains specialist phagocytes (engulfing cells) which remove tiny particles of bone and cartilage as the joints move against each other. The synovial fluid has a pivotal role in preventing the onset of both RA and OA.

Osteoarthritis is the most common form of arthritis in the world. The figures quoted above for the UK and US form a part of a picture, (which according to the WHO), where 10% of men and 18% of women on the Planet have a diagnosis, making OA the 10th most disabling condition in the global North. As the 20th century passed through its final years very few epidemiological (population) studies had been carried out concerning the incidence of OA in the majority world. Those that have any scientific validity were all carried out on African populations. It is well established that OA is less frequent in the global South and the reasons for this occurrence are as complex as the convoluted story of Life on Earth itself. Since the 1980's similar research on the prevalence of OA has established that the disease is the fourth most debilitating condition in the world. However, across the global south (Africa, Asia, Latin America) and in particular Asia the incidence of OA is rising due to the realities of having a progressively ageing population. Additionally, OA has long been associated with excessive amounts of physical work which in combination with the complete lack of labour laws that we in the West (for now) take for granted, is a perfect negative storm of OA incidence in the majority world. In addition for those individuals with extreme OA in such regions hip and joint replacement surgery is for most of the population as unaffordable as it is inaccessible. Overall, according to the WHO agricultural and physically demanding work increases the risk of developing OA by any value up to a factor of 10, depending on the intensity and type of work carried out. However, as we shall see in chapter four the role of diet and the increase in obesity levels across the board is becoming a source of alarm for rheumatologists. OA is generally associated with ageing but as we shall see in the other book in this series "childhood diseases" it can occur in children and in middle-aged adults and can be induced by injury. OA can strike at any of the joints but the joints of the knees, hips, wrist, fingers and lumbar (lower back) are most susceptible.

OA is a degenerative disease which has particular affinity for the articular (hyaline) cartilage. As the cartilage is worn away it is replaced by new bone and as the ability to move is progressively curtailed.

This situation is exacerbated by the enzymes and cytokines involved in the inflammation response and the result is progressively more intense pain, swelling and joint stiffness. As the hyaline cartilage thins the osteoblasts go into overdrive which actuates the growth of bony protrusions known as osteophytes, which form across the affected joint. The osteophytes form over many years and are the structures responsible for the deterioration of joint movement and so any preventative measure must be shown to have an inhibiting effect on their growth. It is important to stress that the osteophytes themselves are only painful if the impact on the muscular and / or nervous system. However, once the osteophytes start rubbing against each other the joint and therefore the musco-skeletal system will start to deteriorate. The progression of OA is divided into three basic stages. First, the hyaline cartilage as well as metabolism and function of the chondrocyte cells is disturbed. The chondrocytes start to produce a class of enzymes known as metallo-proteinases (only the abstract is necessary but please feel free to read on) which begin to destroy the cartilage as mentioned above. In response the chondrocytes do produce substances called tissue inhibitors of metallo-proteinases (TIMP's) but the quantities are insufficient to mitigate the effect of the metallo-proteinases. A protease is any enzyme which is designed to catalyse the breakup of proteins. For example the proteases in the stomach break down proteins into polypeptides. Stage two of OA is marked by softening, erosion and puncturing of the cartilage surface (fibrillation) and the subsequent release of collagen fragments and connective proteins called proteoglycans, into the synovial fluid. It is the proteoglycans which enable the joint to withstand the physical compresses forces discussed in chapter one. In stage three the breakdown of the cartilage structure and the products of the skewed metabolism of the chondrocytes causes the inflammatory response. The response causes more tissue destruction and /or stimulates the release of extra metallo-proteinase. it is after stage three that the ostephytes are generated.

Several triggers including obesity (and other forms of metabolic imbalance), a concurrent lack of exercise joint injury or wear, genetic or biochemical reasons cause defective cartilage. Generally, once the damaged area measures more than $1cm^2$ the function of the articular cartilage is impaired. This form of arthritis is the major cause of the need for hip and other joint replacement operations. When the social and economic impact of Arthritis is considered the charities involved and the UK NHS do not pull their proverbial punches. For example, as of 2012/13, 11% of the UK population aged 45 has some degree of hip osteoarthritis. In 2013 the NHS budget for treating musco-skeletal conditions exceeded £5.5 billion pounds and as the UK population ages this figure can only increase. Approximately half of this figure is spent on hip replacements or treating hip fractures. By 2036 the figure for hip treatment only, as a whole could well exceed £6 billion. Thus osteoarthritis is a major financial burden to the UK health system and similar assertions can be made across the Western world. As a fundraiser I worked on behalf of an organisation called *"Action on Disability and*

Development". I can only despair at the nightmarish consequences of OA in the majority world. Over 80% of all total hip replacement surgery carried out in the UK is as a result of osteoarthritis. Concurrently, the medical profession is united in its stance that a confluence of ageing, obesity, inactivity and bad diet is the key driver behind the incidence of OA. Hence, it seems fair to assert that although OA cannot be seen as preventable in the same context as type-2 diabetes, it is entirely possible to reduce the risk of developing the diseases by adopting appropriate lifestyle changes.

As was discussed in diabetes inactivity costs the NHS some serious cash, The UK department of health suggests a figure of over £1billion, related to inactivity is the incidence of obesity which adds an additional £5 billion to the figures quoted above. These figures do not serve to partition blame for the funding crisis in the NHS to the population it serves, that is the fault of successive governments and the corporate interests they serve. The point being made throughout this series of books is that we as individuals can do our bit to mitigate such financial impacts of negative health and lifestyle choices. Put simply the onus is on all of us wherever we can to follow the advice put forward in chapter four of this book in particular and the rest of the series in general. Overall in the UK musculoskeletal conditions compose some 30% of the totality of years lived under the shadow of disability. So in terms of arthritis do yourself, your friends and family and in a wider (if simplistic) context the NHS a favour, and follow a balanced non-western diet as much as you can.

As with RA the genetic basis for OA cannot be ignored. In fact one could right several volumes on the genetic basis for the condition and still have room for more. Research published in the UK journal "The Lancet" (amongst other publications) suggests that OA affects 40% of all people aged over 70. By the time we reach our 85th year about half of us will develop the condition. The 2012 study, funded to the tune of over £2million findings further build on our knowledge of the genetic basis for OA. The research compared thousands of patients with severe OA to equivalent numbers of healthy volunteers from four European countries. In short, the findings assert that if both parents have OA then the offspring are twice as likely to develop the disease, particularly in the knee and hip. So the question after genetic, hereditary, age and gender factors are considered is *"what role can diet play in preventing the onset of both RA and OA?"* and so we move on to chapters four and five.

Chapter 4:
Obesity and Arthritis

Let us once again inculcate that there is no treatment which can cure arthritis. So without doubt prevention must play an essential role in removing the health, community, social and personal burdens alluded to in the previous chapter. Any public health initiatives concerning arthritis or conditions such as Type-2 diabetes need to be multi-disciplinary and holistic if they are to stand any chance of success. The good news is that if diagnosed in time OA is not necessarily an inevitable part of getting older and the sooner it is recognised the more likely its progress will be halted. However, it cannot be understated that as we age the risk will increase no matter what risk factors you eliminate. Having said that as with all medical conditions this risk can be reduced if you monitor your Body Mass Index (BMI), undertake appropriate and regular exercise in combination with eating a diet based on fruits, vegetables, pulses, grains and cereals. In other words the proclivity to develop arthritis (and many other negative health conditions) steadily increases in line with an increasing

BMI. In addition the longer the metabolism is out of balance as indicated by your BMI the greater is the chance of developing any one (or more) of said conditions. In terms of arthritis, the greater the BMI the greater is the strain you are placing on a given joint. This is observed particularly in the knee and hip joints, which if you think about it, is pretty self-evident. The other modifiable factor (one that can be controlled) is the level of and type of exercise you partake of. In essence there are clear and direct correlations (in either direction) to the development of arthritis. This chapter will present the evidence as to the role being *"overweight"* or *"obese"* plays in the development of arthritis and will wherever possible be directly linked to the biological processes presented above. The term obesity has been defined elsewhere in this series. At this juncture all that is necessary is to impart that obesity is a condition whereby an individual has accumulated so much fat (adipose tissue) that it is having demonstrable detrimental consequences on their health.

The criticism directed toward the Western Diet has been a constant thread throughout this set of books and so it would seem rude to stop now. As should be apparent this diet is deficient in just about all the nutrients that the body needs whilst being replete with substances that the body can quite frankly do without. Such a diet is the complete antithesis of what has been called the Mediterranean Diet which is rich in legumes, fresh fruits and vegetables, fish and olive oil amongst other wholly desirable foodstuffs.

The *SIRT FOOD* and *diabetes* book's in particular presented plenty of reason why the Western diet should be purged from our culinary culture at the earliest possible convenience. This book uses arthritis as a platform to demand the same level of coordinated individual, local, national and international action. In short the western diet is high in calories, saturated fats, trans-fats (discussed in *diabetes)*, salt, sugar and a whole host of additives. The additives are the substances indicated by capital letters and numbers. In addition we should not be fooled by notions of foods that have been fortified or enriched. Put simply in this context if I have enriched you financially I have taken £20.00 away from you, but given you back £1.00. You wouldn't willingly engage in such a transaction in the real world, so why should you in the equivalent culinary world!

These books are about empowering you the reader to make a choice based on empirical evidence and I certainly do not intend to preach. But I think it can be safe to say the more of a plant based diet full of organic, natural foods the better your chances of preventing inflammatory and degenerate disease. The nutritional value of herbs, spices, ginger and garlic (and many other natural flavorings) resides in their myriad of active compounds whose efficacy is well documented and was indicated in the *"cancer"* book. So sprinkle and season away and the more variety the better. All I'm saying is that you can take control of your diet with a cook book, put some effort in and you're on the way. It really isn't difficult, seriously if I can do it you certainly can. I would certainly recommend growing some of your own organic food, even if it's just a few pots of herbs and a few tomato plants. The avoidance of processes sugar, especially the artificial ones as well as salt (MSG) is tantamount to a healthy constitution. If you want to look after your joints you need to eat all of the vitamins and minerals that best protect them. Along with all the other dietary advice hitherto presented this is achievable if you are eating a genuinely balanced diet. In other words there is no big secret, so get stuck in.

Arthritis is more common in those who are obese and because of the extra mass being carried is particularly prevalent on the knee and hip joints. Putting it bluntly, the more of *"you"* that the joints are supporting the more physical strain they are under. In tandem with the extra mass, adipose tissue (fat cells) is not passive and one metabolic consequence of their existence is the release of biological molecules which promote inflammation. Whilst it is not the subject of this book to discuss the complexity of fatty acid metabolism, it is fair to state that they do contribute to tissue inflammation across the board. This class of chemicals was discussed in the *"SIRT FOOD"* book. Put simply they are a fat molecule which has no extra spaces for other atoms to bond on to. In other words no other atoms of any other element can fit on to the molecule, which is why the term *"saturated"* is employed. You will recognise trans-fats by the term hydrogenated oil on the ingredients list. Hence as can be deduced from the writing above they may well play a role in promoting an inflammatory response. Once again it is various classes of cytokines (cell-signalling molecules) that promote tissue inflammation in obese and overweight persons. Put simply the greater the degree of movement away from an optimal BMI the greater is the degree of release of such biochemical and their release is a direct metabolic consequence of obesity.

Other chemicals implicated in the development of obesity related arthritis include the protein adiponectin (produced by fat cells) and the hormone leptin. Adiponectin is known to promote the insulin resistance intrinsic to type-two diabetes and may have its anti-inflammatory properties suppressed in similar circumstances, particularly in the synovial fluid. However, in terms of arthritis the jury is still deliberating, the reader is invited to peruse this hyperlink (http://bit.ly/1jlKnRQ) for more discussion on adiponectin. As a hormone, leptin controls the appetite by *"telling"* the hormonal control centre of the brain (the hypothalamus) that we are full. The more leptin we have circulating in the blood and endocrine (hormonal) system the less responsive the hypothalamus becomes, such that we feel hungry, even if we are clearly not. Leptin may have an indirect role in the onset of arthritis because its elevated concentration additionally may promote inflammation. In other words leptin has a critical role in communicating information concerning the level of fat in the body. Although RA is generally considered an autoimmune condition its intensity is absolutely exacerbated by the risk factors presented above and so obesity prevention can clearly be viewed as one essential mechanism for preventing the onset of arthritis.

The reader has hopefully by now understood that inflammation is a pre-cursor to arthritis and so the diet has a pivotal role in keeping metabolism in a non-inflamed state. Annex 1 below presents a table of foods to avoid or seriously curtail if you wish to reduce inflammation and lose some weight into the bargain. In other words you are looking to move away from a Western Diet and take control of your eating habits. Which, honestly is so easy, really, it is! The table is presented for indicative purposes and is no way to supersede the professional medical advice from either doctors, dieticians or the team involved in developing any kind of treatment plan. The table also presents an opportunity to inculcate the word balance. An excess of any food stuff is undesirable. For example, we all know the benefits of oils such as omega three and six oils but consuming excessive amounts once again promotes inflammation. Overall these oils are believed to inhibit the production of inflammatory enzymes and promote the production of anti-inflammatory substances. In turn this is a damage reduction exercise in terms of the positive impact on the strength of collagen, cartilage and the connective (tendons and ligaments) tissues they are used to manufacture. As a general rule eat these oils in situ, that is as present in fresh foods as opposed to refined foods, condiments and oils. Artificial sweeteners such as aspartame can be dangerous for a whole host of reasons. Many of these additives are not nutritional, highly processed substances and aspartame is a recognised neuro toxin. Which means it can attack the cells of the brain, central nervous and peripheral nervous systems. Some individuals are particularly sensitive and the immune system becomes tricked into seeing the metabolites as foreign antigens. Overall any diet that reduces inflammation is beneficial to inhibiting the onset of arthritis.

Annex 1 Table Two Foods Which May Promote the Onset of Arthritis

Foodstuff	Consequence
Refined Sugar	Excess is stored as glycogen before conversion to fat
Saturated Fats	Trigger additional inflammation
Trans fats mainly found in fried fast foods	A form of saturated fat and so cause additional inflammation
Excessive amounts of oils (E.g. Omega 3 / 6)	Trigger additional inflammation
Refined carbohydrates – Any white refined food product	High glycemic index (see diabetes) lead to excessive glucose which is converted to glycogen and then fat, leading to inflammation

Alcohol	Metabolism produces fatty acids but overall puts extra strain on the liver, especially if you are already obese. So cut down regardless and watch the units!
Aspartame / MSG – amongst other additives	Can be dangerous regardless, but are implicated in triggering an autoimmune response. MSG is widely thought to affect the liver and promote inflammation pathways
Gluten and Casein	For those with a recognised intolerance reducing inflammation is the key

Chapter 5:
Diet and Arthritis

Chapter four unequivocally states that a balanced diet is essential to mitigating obesity. The principle nutrients believed to be involved in the prevention of arthritis are the B vitamins in their entirety, vitamins C, D, E and K. Trace elements (minerals) such as the non-metal phosphorous, and the metalloid boron as metals including calcium, magnesium iron, zinc, calcium, copper, and selenium. Other important nutrients include anthocyanins a type of flavonoid which was mentioned in the "cancer" book. The flavonoids are a huge family of chemicals which serve the plant by protecting it from the attentions of pathogenic bacteria, viruses, and other microbes. Flavonoids are one family of phytochemicals; these are plant based and biologically active compounds. There are many thousands of phytochemicals and needless to say their collective role in ensuring healthy nutrition is the subject of wide-ranging and detailed research. Whether or not any of these chemicals will specifically help with arthritis is a long way from being established. Lest we forget, human beings need to ingest all twenty amino acids to ensure their metabolic health and well-being but proline is of particular interest for arthritis prevention.

Put simply, with arthritis we are talking about inhibiting the onset of inflammation and so that means a balanced quota of a wide range of anti-inflammatory molecules is essential. As can be inferred from the above writing any foodstuff that aids in growth and support of collagen and muscle fibres is going to mitigate the biological conditions which promote arthritis. In essence, any food which contains the above elements and/ or compounds could play a role in arthritis prevention. A summary of such foods is presented in Annex 2. The Mediterranean diet as discussed elsewhere is the complete nutritional opposite of its Western diet counterpart. The totality of real and potential health benefits of such a diet was made clear in the "*SIRT FOOD*" book, but such attributes have been recognised for several decades. For our purposes, the key point to make is the Mediterranean diets are rich in anti-inflammatory molecules. As chronic inflammation is a definite precursor to arthritis the potential utility of such a diet ought to be obvious. One component of such a diet is its complement of fish such as halibut, sardines, mackerel, herring, salmon, sardines and tuna. These fish are rich in omega 3 and 6 fatty acids, antioxidants and phytochemicals which directly or as they are metabolised supply the body with anti-inflammatory substances.

However, and without preaching, I would be in remiss if I did not make clear the context in which this statement of fact must be placed. The same arguments that can be charged against the meat industry can also without equivocation be laid at the door of the global intensive fishing (well fish mining) industry. The classic example is, of course, the humble Cod and yes I do mean the fish you have that quintessentially British culinary delight we call the *"fish supper"*. In 1968 the Canadian fishing industry was worth approximately 1.5 billion dollars, as of 2015 it is worth some few tens of millions of dollars at best. A definite example of long term planning there then! Sarcastic, me, never! In short, due to grotesque overfishing (mining) and total disregard for the ecology of Atlantic and Pacific fish stocks of cod and other once abundant fish species, numbers have all but collapsed and show little sign of recovery. The story behind the collapse of The Newfoundland Grand Banks fishery is not an isolated case. Cod numbers are now no more than 3% of their previously massive quantities. Such realities are the principle driver behind the recent decision of the Canadian Government to restart the annual harp seal cull, although demand for the infant seal fur itself also contributes. Global stocks of tuna fish now face similar catastrophic decline and overall fish stocks around the world are in dire straits, to put it mildly. Many staple fish (such as Cod) are on the International Union for the Conservation of Nature (IUCN) Red List and face extinction. For instance since the 1970's stocks of bluefin tuna have declined by anything up to 90%, depending on whose statistics you believe. The impact on marine biodiversity really is enough to elicit feelings of disgust and sadness at this kind of environmental crime. None of this is your fault any more than it is mine; the blame lies with the conglomerates which control the global fishing industry.

The point is that you can obtain all of the anti-inflammatory biological molecules you need from a vegan or vegetarian diet. So, this means you can eat fruits, vegetables, nuts, beans, pulses, whole grains, extra virgin olive oil (EVOO) and still assuage arthritis. Alternatively, you can eat fish from certifiable sustainable resources and that means your default position has to be to disbelieve totally anything the supermarkets tell you, at least until you have checked for yourself. Getting back on track the research literature is filled with literally hundreds if not thousands of scientific papers which discuss the anti-inflammatory virtues of a balanced diet. If such a diet improves joint function and so your mobility, reduces any kind of stiffness and overall functionality, then it has to be considered beneficial irrespective of any arthritis preventing credentials. The remainder of this chapter will consider some of the other substances which are widely believed to inhibit inflammation and so could temper the onset of arthritis.

Oleocanthal: Present in high quantities in EVOO and comes from the family of chemicals known as phenols, which are common across the biosphere. Oleocanthal (decarboxy methyl ligstroside aglycone) is a recognized anti-inflammatory and is for our purposes chemically similar to the active ingredients found in Ibuprofen. So, you now have another after dinner talking point and example of a plant based medical product. According to a recent review on the subject, oleocanthal has been shown to have a demonstrable impact on inflammatory pathways that act as precursors to diseases such as arthritis. EVOO has been a dietary staple in the region for thousands of years and Hippocrates apparently listed 60 conditions which could be at least partially treated by EVOO. Overall oleocanthal is but one of dozens (so far discovered) of compounds which are believed to help in the prevention and management of the non-communicable disease. However, it is oleocanthal that is the proverbial *"grande fromage"* and its NSAID (non-steroid anti-inflammatory drug) properties are indeed exceptional. In summary, oleocanthal functions by inhibiting the inflammatory action of two enzymes cyclooxygenase 1 and 2. Furthermore, the action is dose dependent, that is the more that is taken the greater the effect. This does not mean that you should be drinking litres of EVOO every day as that will make you decidedly ill, just use as normal. Overall, further research is needed but the potential for being able to say *"yes oleocanthal can be used to prevent, treat or manage arthritis"* is huge. In addition when eaten in this form the anti-inflammatory properties are expressed without the damaging gastrointestinal side effects of certain prescribed drugs. Hence another two reasons for the price of EVOO to made more affordable for the population.

The B (complex) vitamins: These are vitamins that should form part of your diet as a matter of course (pun intended); they are all water soluble and so not stored by the body. This means the B vitamins must be replaced on a daily basis by eating the foods which contain them. All 8 B vitamins facilitate the conversion of carbohydrates (such as starch) into glucose, which is used in cellular respiration, also your nervous system would seize up without them. In addition, the B complex vitamins help with the digestion, metabolism, and assimilation of fats and proteins, so the liver needs a regular and steady supply. In terms of aesthetic health (how we look) the B vitamins are needed for a healthy looking skin (which is an organ in its own right), eyes and of course our hair. So, *"Beam"*me up Scotty (go on laugh you know you want to)! Ok for arthritis research focuses on vitamin B6 (pyridoxine), B3 (niacin), and B12 (folic acid / folate) as these are the B vitamins (amongst others) that facilitate the mobility and action of the synovial joints. As with vitamins and minerals discussed below no causative link has been established, meaning we cannot say eating a B vitamin will prevent arthritis. What we can say is that research literature focuses on the lack of these vitamins in persons who suffer from arthritis and that for B vitamins the deficiency is more apparent for those suffering from RA.

Vitamin C: Also known as ascorbic acid and has multiple roles in the body. It is water soluble and so must be replenished on a daily basis. The classic symptom of vitamin deficiency is scurvy which amongst other painful or undesirable effects impacts on the ability of the body to manufacture collagen effectively. In effect, less of this essential connective tissue is made and the functionality of what is made is inferior as compared to healthy tissue. In addition, the bones themselves become brittle, ossification and reformation are impaired and the bones do not heal properly. As discussed in the *"SIRT FOOD"* book, vitamin C is a very strong anti-oxidising agent, which helps impair the onset of inflammation. There is some suggestion that as part of a balanced diet vitamin C may play a role in repairing the damage caused by arthritis. Other research suggests that arthritis progresses more rapidly in persons who have a diet deficient in ascorbic acid. Similar findings have been suggested for vitamins D, E, and K but research is a long way from hypothesising any definite link or causative correlation. What we can say is that these vitamins are all good for you because they facilitate so many important biological reactions and ensure that our organ systems function at their optimum level. As a corollary to really feel the benefits one must be following a balanced diet and be monitoring their lifestyle choices at all opportunities, especially if you are in middle age, or older.

A vitamin is any organic (carbon-based) biological molecule which is fat or water soluble which the human body needs to carry out its functions. All animals obtain the vitamins they need from their diet and human beings are no different in this respect. If any one of these vitamins is missing then the person is said to have a vitamin deficiency. In contrast, a mineral is any inorganic (non-carbon-based) substance as exemplified in the opening paragraph. Minerals are absolutely essential for life on Earth, for example, photosynthesis would not be possible without the presence of trace amounts of magnesium inside the molecules of chlorophyll. A comparable level of importance is applicable to human metabolism. For example ions of sodium and potassium are needed to transmit nervous impulses across nerve synapses and calcium ions are needed in the movement of the muscles as well as for bone formation. Again there is no secret to obtaining these elements all that is required is the ingesting of a balanced non-western diet. It must be stressed that metals, when ingested as part of a normal balanced diet, are essential; however, this is not true if the route of ingress is through pollution and or excessive consumption of supplements. In the former case, metals can have severe consequences for the people concerned and metal supplement consumption has been linked many adverse medical effects. So do not consume any mineral supplements unless you are advised to do so as part of a prescribed medical treatment. You can obtain all of the essential minerals you need from a balanced diet. Copper exemplifies this last point perfectly, in the *"cancer"* book some discussion was made on the link between red meat and cancer, so if you're eating red meat keep it to one portion of no more than 500g per week. This will give your body plenty of time to metabolise the meat and reduce any extra strain on your metabolism. The metabolism of iron is another case in point, the jury is still out, but there is evidence that Iron from animal sources is better absorbed than from plant sources. However, this fact is more than outweighed by the proven virtues of a vegetarian / vegan diet. In terms of arthritis, the available information is wide-ranging and detailed · and this hyperlink (http://bit.ly/1VPAPj2) presents is a good jumping off point. Overall, the minerals presented in table one are involved directly in bone ossification or resorption, the synthesis (manufacture) of connective tissues and /or the metabolic and biological processes which transport such elements in the correct form.

Ok, I think the point about diet vitamins, minerals and lots of substances with long chemical names has been made. I could keep going and I could write a book on the efficacy or not on metal such as copper alone. There are dozens of hyperlinks throughout this text and supporting references listed, so please feel to dive in and follow whichever direction you desire, there truly is plenty more that you can contribute.

Annex 1 Table One Foods Which May Help Prevent The Onset Of Arthritis

Substance	Foodstuff
The B vitamins	Wheat germ, Bananas, pulses, mushrooms, spinach, seeds, beans, bran
Vitamin C	Citrus Fruits, Strawberries, Peppers And Broccoli, leafy green (cruciferous) vegetables

Vitamin D	Mustard, oily fish, mushrooms, egg yolk, tofu, cereals, soy, yoghurt
Vitamin E	Nuts, Seeds, Wheat Germ, Spinach, Beet / Root Vegetables, Avocado
Vitamin K	Cruciferous Vegetables, Cold Pressed Oils, Whole Grains, Beet / root vegetables
Calcium	Shellfish, Nuts, Red Meat And Some Potable Water Supplies
Copper	Dark Leafy Cruciferous Vegetables, Dried Fruits, Potatoes, Beans, Nuts, Whole Grains, Liver And Red Meat
Selenium	Brazil nuts, Turkey, whole grains, shrimp, tuna, Chicken
Iron	Pulses, Peas, Raisins, Spinach, Beans, Liver, Beef, Turkey, Fish
Anthocyanin's	Blackberries, Blue Berries, Cherries And Raspberries
Proline	Egg White, Meat, Cheese, Soy And Cabbage
Oleocanthal	Extra Virgin Olive Oil (EVOO)
Omega 3	Oily / Cold water / Certifiably Sustainable Caught Fish
	Herbs, Spices, Ginger, and Garlic

Sources

General Sources

http://www.ncbi.nlm.nih.gov/pubmedhealth/PMHT0022042/

Rheumatoid Arthritis / Osteoarthritis

http://www.allaboutbackandneckpain.com/learn/spinesub_learn.asp?id=200

http://www.arthritis.org/about-arthritis/types/rheumatoid-arthritis/causes.php

http://onlinelibrary.wiley.com/doi/10.1002/art.1780301102/pdf

http://www.hopkinsarthritis.org/arthritis-info/rheumatoid-arthritis/ra-pathophysiology-2/

https://www.qiagen.com/gb/products/genes%20and%20pathways/pathway%20details/?pwid=350

http://www.arthritis-research.com/content/16/2/R61

http://ard.bmj.com/content/60/3/223.full

http://www.ncbi.nlm.nih.gov/pmc/articles/PMC416453/

http://umm.edu/health/medical/reports/articles/osteoarthritis

http://www.who.int/chp/topics/rheumatic/en/

http://www.sanger.ac.uk/about/press/2012/120703.html

http://www.hopkinsarthritis.org/arthritis-info/osteoarthritis/oa-pathophysiology/

http://www.england.nhs.uk/resources/resources-for-ccgs/prog-budgeting/

Obesity and Arthritis

http://www.arthritis.org/living-with-arthritis/comorbidities/obesity-arthritis/fat-and-arthritis.php

http://atvb.ahajournals.org/content/30/4/692.full.pdf+html

Diet and arthritis

http://www.medicalnewstoday.com/articles/7621.php

http://www.arthritis.org/living-with-arthritis/arthritis-diet/anti-inflammatory/eat-to-beat-inflammation.php

http://www.arthritis.org/living-with-arthritis/arthritis-diet/anti-inflammatory/vegan-and-vegetarian-diets.php

http://www.hopkinsarthritis.org/patient-corner/disease-management/role-of-body-weight-in-osteoarthritis/

http://www.ncbi.nlm.nih.gov/pmc/articles/PMC4139846/

http://www.hopkinsarthritis.org/patient-corner/disease-management/rheumatoid-arthrtis-nutrition/

http://www.arthritis.org/living-with-arthritis/treatments/natural/vitamins-minerals/guide/

Useful Website about Health & Nutrition

http://nutritionfacts.org

http://www.naturalnews.com

http://nutritiondata.self.com

https://www.pinterest.com/coco942001/save-yourself/

https://www.pinterest.com/coco942001/clean-food-recipes/

https://viddapublishing.com

http://viddapublishing.blogspot.co.uk/

SIRT FOOD: The Secret Behind Diet, Healthy Weight Loss, Disease Reversal & Longevity

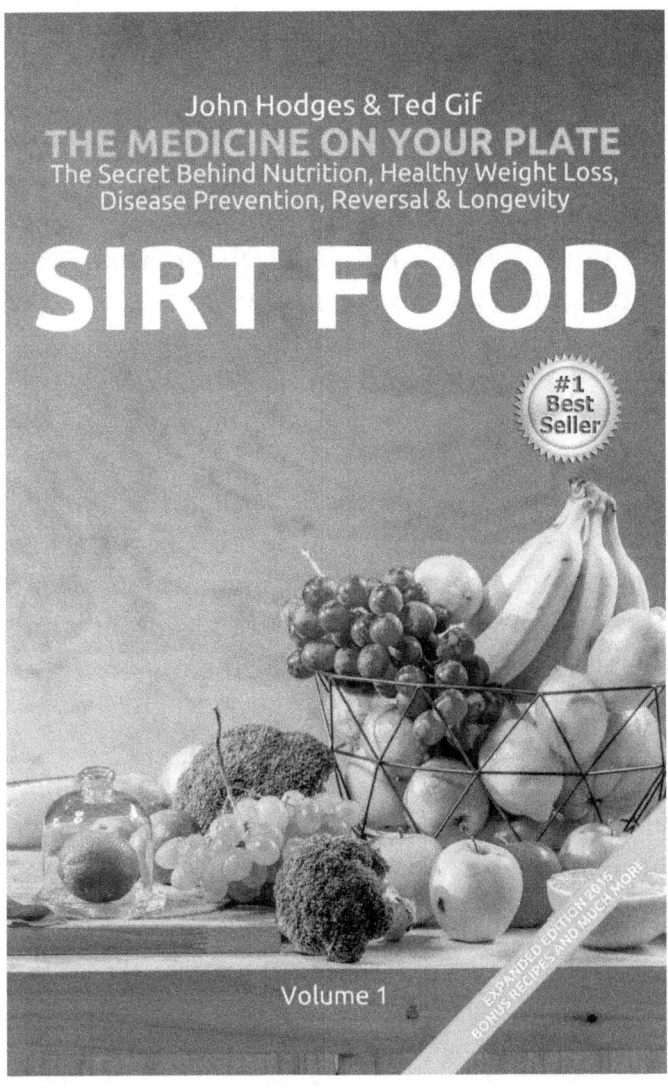

Preface

After the success of SIRTFOOD in 2015/16 hitting #1 in multiple categories on both sides of the Atlantic and ranking high in several foreign markets, we thought it was time for an expanded 2nd edition.

In this updated 2016 edition of SIRT FOOD we are presenting the science, discoveries and a new understanding of these powerful and health restoring proteins. In addition, we explain how these proteins can 'switch on' the DNA in your cells. Therefore strengthening the immune system to help restore health and prevent our most common illnesses and diseases by simply eating the identified and common foods. It's that simple.

Also included is an illustrated section listing the nutrient makeup of our favourite Sirtfoods and some delicious and simple recipes to get you started. These are guides for you to refer to when preparing your meals or in the supermarket choosing which foods to place on your dining table.

In today's modern world, we have a tendency to think that our state of health is governed solely by our genetics and other factors beyond our control. We run to the medical professionals for help and guidance when things go wrong and nine out of ten times we come away unsatisfied with the diagnosis and with an expensive prescription in our hand. Modern medicine has a monopoly on treating symptoms and not addressing the underlying cause of our illness.

Vibrant health depends on many internal and external factors and a ten-minute appointment with your overworked M.D. can be a prescription for a lifetime of reliance on medication and management of their side effects.

Many of our doctors themselves suffer from preventable diseases. I can guarantee most of the readers of this book, at some point in their lives, have visited a doctor and come away thinking "I am in better shape than my doctor is". It's a cliché that the very same doctors handing out statins for high Cholesterol are often squeezed in behind their desks looking like poster boys for obesity, diabetes, addiction, the list goes on.

This work is not in any way a document of criticism of today's advances in modern medicine; far from it. If today, myself or my family needed surgery, whether it be open heart surgery or a hip replacement, I would not hesitate to put my trust and health into their skilled hands. The expertise of our surgeons is undeniable and they save an enhance countless lives every year. Our scientific understanding of the physiology of the human body has never been greater. In the very near future, our surgeons will all be robotic, guided by the mechanical hand with the human surgeon overseeing with incredibly high-resolution Virtual Reality technology. We have a future where optimal human health will be a reality. We'll easily replace worn out parts, grow replacement organs from the individual patient's DNA. No more powerful anti-viral medication to stop the body's rejection of organ transplants. The future of medicine is very exciting; we've come a long way in the last few decades alone.

We are striving for better and more efficient pharmaceuticals with fewer side effects, learning from the natural medicinal molecules we find in nature. But also, saying that, the cost both monetary and on the actual health of the patients can be very high while advancing this field of research. Is this really the best way forward? Every year hundreds of new drugs come into the marketplace promising the ultimate elixir to human health. The almost unbelievable monetary cost to develop, trial and market a new product often creates a conflict of interests (more on this later). We also have the many 'safe' drugs suddenly withdrawn because of patient fatalities and horrible, long-term damage from side effects to the patient. Our society has become a kind of experimental testing ground for many of these drugs. I realise this point of view might be unpopular in certain fields, but the fact is history shows that most pharmaceuticals come at a high price to the patient's health over long term use and the side effect often has to be treated with even more drugs. Could there be a better way?

The key insight of *SIRT FOOD* is that our health is not fixed, but can be constructed by the decisions and choices we make every day, starting with our informed choices we make about our food. The molecules we put into our mouths via our food are the fundamental building blocks for every cell in our bodies. We have a direct route to the integrity and health of our immune system. Our cells need high-grade nutrients to function normally, if we feed them junk and toxins they eventually seek a dire revenge on us for neglecting them. The science is in and a new way of thinking is revolutionising our understanding of the connections between Health & Nutrition. Do we wait for our Doctors to retrain and pass this information onto us? Shockingly most medical professionals have little or no training in nutrition. I've had doctors confess to me that in the course of 10yrs+ training they were lucky to get two weeks on rudimentary nutrition. This explains a lot. Our doctors are trained to apply band-aids over symptoms of illness via pharmaceutical. Here's a quick fix, now go about your day. Very little is ever taught to our society about prevention of disease, and believe or not, the majority of diseases are preventable. We should no longer hand over the responsibility of our health to other people. I hope this book will enlighten you, the reader, to do more research, share the information and take proactive measures with your diets and environments. The acceptance of chronic disease is not acceptable anymore, we can and we will do things better.

The bottom line is, the person responsible for your health is you. 'The Medicine *is* on your Plate', if you choose so.

J. Hodges. November 2016

Introduction

"Out of clutter, find simplicity. From discord, find harmony. In the middle of difficulty lies opportunity"
Albert Einstein

It is probably fair to say that most of us have never heard of the term Sirtfood and to be fair there is no reason why we should have. This book is not an exhaustive analysis or even partial critique of the biology of Sirtfoods or the proteins they are hypothesised to activate. It is more to impart that eating Sirtfoods is not a fad and that the action of SIRT proteins is the subject of detailed research by agencies which are engaged in seeking solutions to conditions ranging from cancer to Alzheimer's disease. You do not need a biology degree to understand what is written herein. However, by necessity there are several key terms that must be explained. I have attempted to deconstruct these explanations and include hyperlinks to certain definitions which are relevant to the subject in hand. I hope the writing generates the enthusiasm to follow up on any "oh I didn't know that" moments that may (or may not) present themselves as you read through the chapters contained in this book. The writing here is aimed at a non-specialist audience (I myself am no expert in this field), who have at least a passing interest (no matter the reason), in understanding some of what happens to the food we eat when it is digested and the power of this to change our health. The reader will come across familiar terms such as healthy living or healthy eating, but will I hope to gain an appreciation of what these terms mean from a biochemical or metabolic perspective. The book is designed to inform, empower and provoke additional enthusiasm for getting back into the kitchen and take full control of your health via nutrition. As will be imparted repeatedly you do not need to reinvent the culinary wheel. In all probability you may just need to give your current wheel an extra impetus. It is hoped that the reader will be inspired to take more control over the food that they eat and maintain an interest in any future developments in the field of SIRT protein research. The essential message of this writing is to encourage further thought, discussion and provoke individual action on the role of a balanced diet on maintaining your own health. However, it is hoped that the reader gains an understanding of the systemic context in which terms such as the "obesity epidemic" are framed. Finally, this is not a book designed to preach it is a book designed to educate. So don't feel you have to read it as a novel, you can flip and skim as you see fit. Get stuck in and comments are duly welcome.

Chapter 1: Introducing Cells, Proteins and Sirtfoods

"Our bodies are our gardens – our wills are our gardeners." William Shakespeare

In essence, a healthy metabolism means that all of your different cell types are functioning as they should. In recent years the role of Sirtfoods and Sirtuin Activators (SA's) in maintaining this healthy function has been the subject of dozens if not hundreds of individual scientific papers. The Silent Information Regulator (SIR) proteins themselves are proteins found in and around cell organelles, they exist, they are real and they are known to have a wide range of functions. This book is going to ask one fundamental question, *"Is there any credence to the notion that eating Sirtfoods can influence the activity of the SIRT proteins?"* To begin answering this question we must outline some of the biology of living cells, this will take a few sentences. Cells are the building blocks of all living organisms and the organisation of individual cells into organs and organ systems enables complete organisms to function independently in their environment. The organelles are the individual structures situated between the outer cell membrane and the inner nuclear membrane of the cell. The former membrane separates the cell contents from its external environment and controls the movement of nutrients into the cell and the removal of the waste products of metabolism. For example in respiration, oxygen and glucose are transported into the cell and the waste product carbon dioxide is removed. The nuclear membrane separates the cell cytoplasm and organelles from the nucleic acids (such as DNA) situated in the nucleus. The organelles include structures such as the mitochondria, ribosomes and Golgi apparatus. Each organelle is found in a fluid medium called the cytoplasm which is contained between the nuclear and cell membranes. Each organelle is surrounded by an exceptionally thin layer of fluid called the cytosol. The proteins themselves are a hugely diverse and absolutely essential class of biological molecules. Think of any biological or metabolic process and it is more than likely that a protein is involved. They are found in all living organisms and contain different arrangements of atoms of carbon, hydrogen, oxygen as well as nitrogen and some also contain sulphur. The term protein is derived from the Greek word *"prota"* which means *"of primary importance"*. Over two million individual proteins exist in an adult human being and each has a specific task. However, many also have additional functions.

Sirtuin proteins are known to play a crucial role in regulating biochemical processes such as the cell cycle and cell reproduction. In short the SIRT proteins are widely believed to have a profound influence on metabolism in general. In biology the term *"metabolism"* refers to the totality of biochemical reactions which make life possible. At the time of writing there are 7 known SIRT proteins, which are imaginatively tagged as SIRT1 to SIRT7. Without inferring any sense of priority, SIRT1 has by far been the subject of most research on the entire subject of Sirtfoods and their biochemistry. SIRT1 is widely believed to regulate the life cycles of many living cells and is also thought to influence the action of the hormone (amongst others) insulin, promote the breakdown of subcutaneous fat and regulate the tolerance to essential molecules such as glucose. At the outset it is probably helpful to impart that studies suggesting that SIRT1 as an agent of longevity have been seriously questioned by the scientific community. The subtleties pertaining to the term *"longevity"* will be addressed throughout the text and in the section hyperlinked above. Overall, the corpus of knowledge concerning Sirtfoods and the Sirt proteins themselves imparts that their activity is holistic and inter-related. When one considers their distribution within the cell, this assertion should not be surprising. Table one shows the primary location of each Sirt protein but the reader should be aware that each can be found elsewhere in the cytosol and/or cytoplasm of the cell. In addition the possible benefits are derived from studies involving laboratory animals. For example, SIRT 2 is thought to have a role in extending the life span of individual yeast cells but has to date not demonstrated an equivalent action in human beings.

Table 1 introducing the 7 (known) Sirt Compounds (Sirtuin Activators)

Name of Sirt Protein	Primary Location in the Cell	Possible metabolic Benefits
SIRT 1	Nucleus	Metabolism and respiration including promoting mitochondria formation. Enhanced brain function, alertness and cognisance.
SIRT 2	Cytosol	Unclear but is found mainly (but not exclusively) in

		the neurones of the brain. Possible role in mitosis and regulating aging.
SIRT 3	Mitochondria	Regulates respiration. May influence cell aging and reduce tumor formation.
SIRT 4	Mitochondria	Regulates respiration, the action of insulin and fat metabolism.
SIRT 5	Mitochondria	Regulates respiration and stimulates certain enzymes. Structural repair of other Sirt proteins.
SIRT 6	Nucleus	Unknown but has strong correlations to controlling the symptoms of aging.
SIRT 7	Nucleus	Confirmed role in ribosome

		formation DNA replication and protein synthesis. May inhibit tumour formation.

Defining the SIRT proteins

SIRT1: Known to have a role in a wide range and increasing number of functions. Overall research focuses on how the compound functions and mediates in conditions which include obesity, cancer, cardiovascular and pulmonary (heart and lung) disease, dementia and stress.

SIRT2: Interest in this Sirt protein stems from the fact that it is in fact the mammalian equivalent of a protein known as Sir 2, which is found in yeast. This substance potentially has a role in tumour suppression, regulating mitosis (cell division) as well as the copying and synthesis of nucleic acids. It is thought to be a key determinant of the rate at which cells age.

SIRT3: The main focus of SIRT 3 research is its possible role as an inhibitor of tumour growth and hence is of particular interest to oncologists (scientists who study cancer). However, it may well also have a role in the stress response and so can additionally be framed as having importance in that area. Overall SIRT3 may have more importance for cancer, longevity and overall metabolic function in the male of the species.

SIRT4: Once again oncologists are interested in SIRT4 due to its apparent tumour suppressing properties. However, it also has a role in responding to nucleic acid damage, including to DNA. Researchers have additionally shown that SIRT4 regulates fatty acid oxidation in the liver and muscle cells and so could have a role in the treatment of obesity and type-2 diabetes. It is known to suppress the release of insulin from the pancreas if DNA is damaged or if the concentration of amino acids becomes too high in the blood stream. In organisms with a reduced SIRT4 level the incidence of genetic instability (mutations) increases markedly.

SIRT5: The dominant role for SIRT5 is thought to be in regulating the processes which remove ammonia and other toxins from the body via the urea cycle that is through the kidneys, renal system and liver. It is also thought to have a strong function in regulating the rate at which energy is transferred through living cells and respiration in general.

SIRT6: Perhaps underlining the importance of the sirtuins, SIRT6 is thought to be involved in the processes which govern the onset of aging. Additionally, it is known to be involved in the repair of DNA and associated structures as well as the breakdown of glucose molecules (glycolysis) and may contribute to the immune response by regulating inflammation.

SIRT7: There is a very strong body of research which indicates that SIRT7 has an important role in the transcription (copying of DNA). To complicate the work of oncologists, reduced levels of SIRT7 are known to inhibit the growth of tumors. In addition SIRT 7 may well be integral to the effective functioning, maintenance and construction of the ribosomes, which are the site of protein synthesis (manufacture) in a living cell.

A Sirtfood is any food stuff that is able to act as a source of the chemicals (nutrients from food) which stimulate Sirt protein activity. All proteins are coded for by the action of specific sequences of De-oxy Ribonucleic Acid (DNA). In other words each Sirt protein is coded for by a different gene within the molecules of DNA found in the nucleus of our cells. As can be deduced from the data presented above the precise mode of action of the sirtuins in human beings is not fully understood. However, we do know that they are enzymes and as such will be of prime importance to maintaining, regulating and otherwise influencing biochemical reactions. For example SIRT5 is known to directly control at least 700 individual proteins. From here it is fair to propose that in their entirety the sirtuins probably modulate several thousand metabolic processes. If the nucleic acids such as DNA control the biology of an organism then it may be helpful to view the sirtuins as intermediaries, in that the SIRT proteins act on the biochemical instructions passed on to them by DNA. For a food to be considered an SA it must be shown to enhance the rate at which the SIRT enzymes carry out their function. There are many thousands of individual enzymes and they all have a unique function and as a class of biological molecules they are absolutely essential to life as we know it. All enzymes accelerate the rate at which a specific biochemical (metabolic reaction) occurs, with the enzyme undergoing no chemical change in the process. Hence enzymes are often referred to as biological catalysts. For example, every single cell in every single living human being has a nucleus, except for red blood cells. In the early stages of the red blood cell cycle, the cell does possess a nucleus but over time this is substituted for the protein haemoglobin and the enzyme carbonic anhydrase. The blood vessels of the body are organised such that every single cell receives all the nutrients it needs and that all waste products are removed. In red blood cells haemoglobin carries oxygen to our approximately *forty trillion* cells and carbonic anhydrase catalyses the reaction that converts Carbon Dioxide - CO_2 (a waste product of respiration) into hydrogen carbonate. The hydrogen carbonate breaks down in the alveoli of the lungs and the CO_2 is expelled. Without carbonic anhydrase the CO_2 produced in respiration would rapidly build up becoming toxic and you would die from CO_2 poisoning very quickly indeed! In the human organism there are hundreds of different types of cell and each has a precise structure and function. Overall the thrust of research on SIRT proteins concerns their role (or not) in equally important processes and as a corollary the fundamental question asked in the opening paragraph.

The SA's are derived from various food stuff which includes leafy green vegetables such as kale, green tea and extra virgin olive oil. It gets better! If like me you are partial to a glass of vino, then you're in luck because red wine is believed to contain known SA's. Ditto if you like apple crumble, juice or its alcoholic variant, we know as cider! Furthermore, if you're partial to the occasional curry or meat, lentil or spicy bean burgers (or combinations thereof) then don't spare the turmeric. Until recently turmeric was an important dye, but was superseded by synthetic alternatives derived from the petrochemical industry. This versatile and distinctly coloured herbaceous powder has long been used in Asian cookery. Aside from providing you with a quick and easy source of the compounds which are considered to be SA's, turmeric will give your food an extra boost. Not to be outdone lovers of chocolate can rest assured that a moderate intake of a high cocoa confection will boost your SA count. Finally, citrus fruits contain SA's, so instead of buying a carton of processed juice, get yourself a few oranges and squeeze them yourself. There is very little difference in cost and the taste of freshly squeezed orange juice is a different league to its concentrate derived and packaged counterpart.

Provided your diet is balanced eating foods which are high in SA's will not require any major radical change to your eating habits. For instance, I make an allowance to add kale or spinach to the sauces and soups that are regularly concocted in our kitchen. If I am making a salad then it will almost certainly have olives added and a good pokey dressing based on mustard and olive oil will be on hand for drizzling purposes. If you are making a fruit dessert or smoothie you can boost your Sirt credentials by adding blue berries and / or black currants. Having Pie and mash potato? Then add some chopped parsley with the milk, salt, pepper and mustard and work that masher as normal. If you are unsure of a side dish why not try a portion of braised greens including kale. Parsley can also be sprinkled on omelettes which from a Sirtfood perspective ought to contain olives and onions amongst the entirety of lovely fresh vegetables bound together by your mustard, pepper and herb flavoured eggs. In other words eating Sirtfoods as a normal part of a healthy balanced diet should not present most of us with any problems. In fact it would be fair to say that we are already consuming some Sirtfoods and that the only necessary point to make is that you may need to add a few more to your diet. If variety is the spice of life, then the kitchen is included, so why not experiment?

I probably shouldn't say that using fresh juices such as from black currants or red grapes to concoct your favourite tipple adds a whole new dimension to the term *"mixer"*. Oops! I've done it now; there is no going back, oh well! You better drink responsibly. In general research has yet to ascertain the precise mechanisms by which the sirtuins are activated by the chemicals present in Sirtfoods. Concurrently, it cannot as yet be categorically stated how any such activation will express itself in human beings. For example, the scientific literature contains research which asserts that the compound resveratrol may reduce the formation of the plaque in laboratory mice which have been genetically engineered to express the proteins believed to be implicated as a cause of Alzheimer's disease. The degree to which resveratrol displays the same results (if at all), has yet to be established in human suffers from Alzheimer's disease or indeed other forms of dementia such as CJD. Overall the totality of research on the efficacy of Sirt proteins on human beings (and other higher mammals) asserts that they have a non-specific and diverse range of functions. OK assuming you're still reading, let's get on with it and get things rolling by asking *"what are we talking about here?"*

Chapter 2: What is a Sirtfood or MediterrAsian Diet?

"The Chinese do not draw a distinction between food and medicine" Lin Yutang (1895 – 1976) writing in The Importance of Living

A diet rich in Sirtfoods is also known as a (MediterrAsian) diet so named after the geographic regions in which these foods are consumed as a matter of course (the pun is 100% intended). Both Asian and Mediterranean diets are characterised by prolific consumption of fresh fish and legumes, cereals, fruit as well as non-leguminous vegetables. Dairy consumption is moderate and meat especially red meat is very low and as such the MediterrAsian diet is the complete antithesis of what is referred to in nutritional circles as the *"western diet"*. In other words the western diet is high in dairy and meat products, refined sugars and saturated fats as well as being characterised by processed and pre-packaged foods. Perhaps underlying its culinary importance the Mediterranean diet was recognised in 2013 by UNESCO as being of "intangible cultural heritage" in many Mediterranean countries. Coincidentally, in the same year, the New England Journal of Medicine published research which appears to support what we have all been told for decades. Namely, that a diet which is rich in fresh fruit and vegetables and low in fats is good for you. The above study spent 30 years following a cohort of 7,500 Spaniards aged between 55 and 85 years, split roughly equally between genders who consume the Mediterranean diet. In scientific circles it is rare to come across such succinct and direct conclusions. The interdisciplinary team of researchers state that there is an *"absolute risk reduction"* in the incidence of cardiovascular emergencies such as stroke and coronary heart disease as well as heart attacks. The research then clearly states that following the Mediterranean diet reduces the risk of such emergencies by almost a third. Without a doubt this type of primary research gives empirical evidence in support of consuming a diet which is of the MediterrAsian composition. It is important to stress that the researchers involved did not advocate or approve of terms such as *"superfood"*. Furthermore, there is no suggestion the diet would be a substitute for a proscribed medical treatment. In fact it was recommended to participants (in the strongest possible terms), that all such treatments should continue. However, in terms of a preventative measure that can be easily integrated into a person's lifestyle choices the evidence is more than compelling. In fact too many people think such findings represent a succinct definition of the term *"self-evident"*.

In this particular study weight loss or longevity were not the subjects of study and individuals were not given strict menu regimes or generally required to count the calories. In short participants were allowed a bit of *"what they fancy"* as long as they kept to the overall dietary requirements necessary to participate in the study. In the world of Sirtfoods you are not sticking to a strict dietary regime with an equally punishing exercise schedule. You are following a healthy balanced diet plus a few necessary extras, washed down by the occasional treat. In this particular study only 7% of participants dropped out within two years but in contrast 14% of people dropped out in the part of the study where diet was much more proscriptive. This is good news because it should impart that anyone can follow a diet rich in Sirtfoods provided they make a little effort and of course keep improving their cooking skills. The research did acknowledge the cost of certain ingredients such as extra virgin oil which does cost more than other types of olive oil. The difference isn't much, but if you're on a budget every penny counts and so in the real world cost is a factor.

Whether they intended to or not, to acknowledge this fact the scientists involved provided participants with extra virgin oil and any other ingredients as necessary to keep them on board. Having stated that, it is equally important to stress that the foods mentioned below are affordable, have proven nutritional benefits and are easy to incorporate into your diet if you are spending time in the kitchen; that is not just at parties. The next section provides an overview of the principle Sirtfoods, their vitamin and mineral content as well as any information pertaining to the SIRT proteins the food may activate. It is important to realise that the properties outlined below are not an exhaustive list and the reader is encouraged to follow up on any stand of information presented as they see fit. The reader should also be aware that many of the substances discussed are present in more than one food. Finally, the benefits presented below should be viewed from a perspective where the person is not undergoing any prescribed medical treatment. The points made should only impart that eating these food stuff can be easily integrated into any balanced diet and are in no way a substitute for advice from your doctor or dietitian.

Black Currants and Blue Berries:

Aside from tasting absolutely incredible blue berries are a rich source of polyphenol compounds, the particular type being named anthocyanin. Now, you do not need to know the precise chemical structure or even make up of this family of organic (carbon based) chemicals. You do need to appreciate that polyphenol are highly efficient anti-oxidants and so help the cell resist damage from what is termed Cellular Oxidative Stress (COS), which is outlined in the section on **free radicals.** Anthocyanin has been shown to protect laboratory animals from neurological damage and improve their cognitive functions. In clinical (human) trials anthocyanin has been shown to improve the memory function of older adults suffering from dementia. Further research imparts that a preventative function for anthocyanin is more likely if food stuff such as blueberries is consumed regularly and as part of a normal balanced diet. Overall blue berries are a high density source of anti-oxidants, vitamins such as A, C, and E as well as essential trace elements such as selenium, potassium, copper, iron and manganese. Blue berries are an important source of the B vitamins which are known to facilitate the metabolism of the three principle types of biological molecules (fats, proteins and carbohydrates). Ok so you get the point, blue berries are good. In terms of SIRT protein research continues but the anti-oxidants present are thought to promote the action of SIRT1 and SIRT 2. In general terms black currants are believed to express equivalent health benefits.

Green Tea:

Green tea is native to India and China where its health benefits have been recognised for centuries, it is the unrefined form of the more familiar black tea and accounts for about 20% of all the tea that is consumed globally. Green tea is well known to contain more anti-oxidants, such as polyphenols than its black and more processed counterpart. For example a polyphenol known as epigallocatechin-3-gallate (EGCG) is according to some medical researchers the polyphenol most associated with preventing the incidence of tumours. Helpfully ECGC is one of many key active polyphenols in green tea. A cursory google search will present the corpus of knowledge that indicates a chemo-preventative role for ECGC in laboratory animals and it may even help the body cope with chemotherapy. In addition epidemiological (people) studies have shown some reduction in the risk of cancers of the stomach, colon, blood vessels, skin, prostate gland, bladder, lungs, the breasts (mammary glands) and oesophagus. In terms of cancer prevention ECGC is thought to function by suppressing the factors which allow cancer cells to develop in the first instance. Overall medical research suggests that ECGC has great potential for the treatment of disease, particularly cancer in homo-sapiens this should not be surprising due to the pedigree which the green tea plant possesses. In traditional medicines green tea leaves are used to treat wounds, improve the functioning of the heart and mental faculties and in the diet it is known to help digestion, it may even help with thermo-regulation (science speak for maintaining an optimum body temperature). In terms of the biology of the Sirtuin proteins, green tea is believed to stimulate the proteins involved in metabolism and may contribute to effective treatment for type-2 diabetes. Additionally, green tea is known to contain *"anti-inflammatory agents"* and could very well promote the activity of all 7 Sirt proteins. Green tea is also a rich source of vitamin K, folic acid and Fluoride.

Dark Chocolate And Cocoa:

Right, shall we get something straight right away; the health benefits outlined here are not meant to signal that you can go to the nearest corner shop and gorge yourself on processed chocolate. We are talking here about a cocoa content and put simply the purported health benefits apply more to the cocoa beans themselves and not to the confection. So seek out high cocoa content chocolate that exceeds 70%, contains no refined sugar, few if any additives or added fats. Limited research exists which implies that cocoa may reduce blood pressure and therefore may have a role treating hypertension as well as maintaining a healthy cardiovascular system. However, this is by no means a certainty and the same can be said for research which suggests cocoa may have a role in preventing bowel (colon) cancer. There are equivalently strong research findings which suggest that cocoa may inhibit the action of stress hormones, but once again the actual scientific basis for the assertion is far from being established. However, the presence of compounds known as flavonoids which are another class of organic compounds related to the poly phenols, implies effective anti-oxidant properties. The flavonoids are also present in green tea, black tea, fruits, berries and thankfully red wine, so cheers! In its totality unrefined cocoa beans contain over 400 biologically active chemicals amongst them is the amino acid tryptophan. At this juncture I'm afraid we need to introduce some more biology!

In total there are 20 amino acids and they are the building blocks for all the proteins in existence. All of the two million (or thereabouts) proteins in the human body and the millions more which exist across the biosphere are made from the same 20 amino acids. Each protein is made (synthesised) in the cell organelle we name the ribosome. The really clever part is that our DNA ensures that each protein is made with an exact and precise order of amino acids, but the not so clever part is that human beings (along with other species of mammal) need to ingest the amino acids we need to manufacture proteins. We acquire these amino acids from proteins, which must first be eaten and digested. In other words the amino acids we use to synthesise proteins were (whether plant or animal) once part of the protein structure of another organism. Tryptophan has an affinity for an enzyme called tryptophan hydrolase which helps assemble tryptophan into the neurotransmitter (a substance which transfers nerve signals from one nerve cell to another) serotonin (amongst others). Hence it follows that amino acids are essential for the effective functioning of the brain and from here we can impart that effective protein synthesis is dependent on healthy ribosomes. If the SIRT proteins in their entirety are essential for healthy metabolism then it may be established that for SIRT7 to be effective on the ribosomes, the other SIRT proteins must have the metabolic conditions in which to function effectively. It is entirely possible that any number of the active chemicals contained within cocoa beans could well be SA's, however it cannot be stressed enough, that this notion is far from being demonstrated. For now enjoy real chocolate as part of a healthy living program and remember that you just don't know what future benefits may present themselves.

Olives and Extra Virgin Olive Oil:

Arguably, the food most associated with the Mediterranean region is the green and black oval shaped fruit from the *Olea Europaea* tree. Since the time of Ancient Greece the olive tree has been the symbol of peace and cooperation because the substances contained in the fruit and the oils derived from it are so essential to a diet built around healthy living. As such the *O.Europea* tree has been valued for thousands of years both as a store of energy in the form of essential fats and for its high concentration of anti-oxidants. Olives are the source of oleocanthal and oleurpein which are recognised as very powerful natural anti-oxidants and along with high concentrations of carotenoids are certainly wonderful drops of good stuff, which may additionally help the body combat diseases ranging from cancer to diabetes to dementia. However, it is unlikely that terms such as "*anti-oxidant*" were used to describe their importance until comparatively recently, I mean oxygen wasn't even discovered until the late 18th century, well 1774 to be precise! Olives contain mono unsaturated fats such as oleic and palmitoleic acid which is known to lower levels of molecules termed low density lipo-proteins (LDL). At this juncture it is crucial that the reader understands that despite the bad press cholesterol is actually essential for healthy metabolism. It is synthesised in the liver and ingested via the consumption of animal fats, in the body cholesterol is used in the manufacture of hormones, aids in the stability of the cell membrane. In digestion enzymes in the liver convert cholesterol into some of the acidic substances which make up bile an important digestive fluid stored in the gall bladder. As part of the digestive process fats are broken in the ileum which is the later part of the small intestine, where fats are emulsified. In essence, bile is secreted from the gall bladder into the ileum and the fats are mechanically broken down into smaller droplets. Emulsification of fats provides a larger surface area upon which the lipase enzymes can catalyse the reactions which break down fats into fatty acids. When this process finishes the bile acids are absorbed back into the blood stream and transported back to the glass bladder and re-used. In short the body does not need very much if any extra cholesterol, it can manufacture enough from the food we eat. Hence if you are eating too much animal fat cholesterol can build up in the blood stream and so the LDL's come into play and carry to sites of deposition, which include but are not limited to the walls of the arteries. In general terms the more cholesterol being carried and deposited by LDL's the greater is the likelihood of serious trauma such as a heart attack. In contrast High Density Lipo-proteins (HDL) work in the opposite direction that is they carry cholesterol from sites of deposition to the liver, where it is broken down into soluble substances and any waste products expelled. Any food such as olives and extra virgin oil which is rich in mono-unsaturated fats promotes the action of HDL's over that of LDL's hence reducing the probability of Atherosclerosis and of suffering from a heart attack induced by Coronary Heart Disease (CHD).

The oils contained within the (not so) humble olive also have anti-inflammatory properties and themselves contain high concentrations of vitamin E (alpha-tocopherol), which is lipid (fat) soluble and plays a crucially important role in holding cell membranes together. Vitamin E also has a role in the free radical clean up discussed below. Just in case you weren't feeling healthy enough olives also contain plenty of trace metallic elements such as zinc, calcium, copper, iron and manganese as well as a smattering of B vitamins including niacin, pantothenic acid and choline. Finally, I am always arguing with my wonderful girlfriend on the virtues of purchasing *"extra virgin"* as opposed to *"olive oil"*. The former is cold pressed and so loses none of the nutrients and essential substances discussed above, more importantly it comes as nature intended because to meet the designation "extra virgin" it must not be processed in anyway shape or form. In terms of Sirtuin Activation the substances locked up inside both green and black olives could promote the action of any Sirt protein involved in regulating anti-oxidant activity, respiration and mitochondrial function, influencing the onset of the symptoms of ageing as well as the rate of fatty acid breakdown.

Kale:

Although phrases such as "superfood" ought to be taken with the proverbial pinch of salt kale would certainly fit into the category. Kale of one type or another has been eaten for thousands of years. This nutritionally dense leafy green vegetable contains vitamins A, K and C as well as trace minerals including manganese and potassium (amongst others), in short you could do very well in the healthy living stakes by eating kale on a regular basis. Kale also contains many of the B vitamins as well as non–metallic elements such as phosphorus. As if that wasn't good enough kale is also an important source of linoleic acid, which is one of the omega-3 fatty acids and all of this is combined with a very low calorie count. Kale continues to get better, as it has a very high concentration of the anti-oxidants which belong to both the polyphenol and flavonoid classes of organic compounds. The two principle flavonoids are the compounds quercetin and kaempferol, but taken together the anti-oxidant credentials of Kale means that it may have an essential role in promoting cardiovascular health, reducing blood pressure as well as being anti-inflammatory, anti-viral and it may have a role in suppressing the spread and growth of tumours. The kale plant contains substances such as sulforaphane and many others which have been shown to inhibit the growth and spread (metastasis) of cancer cells in laboratory animals; however, there is no clear cut evidence of the same processes occurring in human beings. In terms of the reduction of cardiovascular disease kale has the same broad spectrum of benefits concerning the lowering of LDL's as the fats contained within olives and cold pressed olive oil.

Now then! Here is another idea for your kitchen, steam your vegetables! The reason is simple if you boil for too long many of the nutrients will pass out into the water, I mean why else does it take on the colour of the food you are cooking. I suppose you can keep the cooking water as stock, but if you steam significantly less nutrient loss occurs in the first place. Hence, steaming vegetables means more lovely nutrients with long unpronounceable names will be able to fulfil their function in your body as compared to boiling them. In terms of its Sirt credentials kale contains many of the chemical families that have been associated with the efficacy of SIRT proteins so it seems reasonable to postulate that in general terms eating kale could be beneficial. However, more research will be needed before any definite association can be asserted. One area of research is the relationship between sulforaphane and the mechanisms by which it stimulates the enzymes which break down carcinogens.

(Useful video) http://nutritionfacts.org/video/second-strategy-to-cooking-broccoli

Parsley:

Parsley is native to the Mediterranean and has been used for thousands of years as both an herbal medicine and as an accompaniment which improves the flavour and aesthetics of many dishes. The scientific name of the herb is *Petroselinum crispum* and has been confused with coriander more times than I care to mention. It is now used all over the world and is rich source of Vitamin K, C and A in addition to the anti-oxidants outlined elsewhere in this chapter. One of the anti-oxidants present in parsley is a flavonol called Myricetin which has been shown to have demonstrable chemo-preventative impact on skin cancer. The term chemo prevention refers to any therapy or prophylactic (preventative treatment) that uses naturally occurring (normally plant based) compounds or their manufactured counterparts to prevent or treat a cancer. At this juncture it is important to note that the medical professionals in the field do not consider cancer to be a single disease. According Cancer Research UK over 200 different types of cancer have been diagnosed and each has a different and precise mode of action. In the world of cancer research and treatment the role of diet in cancer prevention is receiving more and intense scrutiny from those who are seeking to cure this terrifying disease. Other foods which contain high levels of Myricetin include sweet potatoes, black currants and cranberries. Myricetin is also of interest to those scientists interested in the treatment of type 2 diabetes because of its potential in promoting insulin activity (i.e. the formation of glycogen). In terms of Sirt activation parsley contains many of the substances that are discussed elsewhere in this section and the same can be said for the other recognised Sirtfoods.

The other Sirtfoods are turmeric, capers (an essential ingredient for tartar sauce), citrus fruits, apples, red grapes, red wine, onions, tofu, soya, Miso soup and loveage. All of these foods contain to varying degrees the vitamins, minerals and other substances which are thought to be involved in SIRT protein activation. Some SA's will be present in higher concentrations in one food as compared to another. For example, we cannot categorically state that Miso soup (an all its variants) is a greater SIRT protein activator than say turmeric because we simply do not know. However, given the expanding amount of research on the subject it is only a matter of time before such assertions will be made. How long will this take? Well how long is a piece of string? The reader should not see this as an issue or stumbling block, in fact quite the opposite. Suppose it was established that Miso soup activated SIRT7 and turmeric or loveage activated SIRT3. There is no problem here all you would do is add say loveage to your soup as a garnish and perhaps add turmeric to the risotto you are having for your main evening meal tomorrow night. Said Risotto should also contain onions, parsley and be served with a salad rich in olives and drizzled with extra virgin olive oil. As will be said again and again and again, the keyword is balance. The essential point of this chapter is to make clear that it is not necessary to partake of dietary supplements (unless you have been advised to do so by your doctor). Furthermore, the reader should conclude that all of these foods have a preventative role in mitigating conditions ranging from diabetes to cancer, they are not cures. However, in terms of healthy living there is no substitute for taking control of your diet and that means informing and educating yourself. In a very real sense this chapter should be viewed as a signpost to healthy eating habits. So, to answer this chapter titular question a Sirtfood diet is one which encourages you take control of what you are eating and how you cook your food. It allows you to add a wide range of readily available ingredients to your diet in a creative and interesting way. It enables you to tick all of your nutritional boxes without breaking the bank. It means you can cook amazing food for yourself, friends, family and loved ones quickly as well as improving and expanding your culinary expertise. Oh and it could well improve your biochemistry and keep you out of hospital for a few more years, which sounds like a plan to me! In its entirety, ingesting Sirtfoods dovetails with eminent synergy to notions of following a balanced diet. Unfortunately, it is not as easy as it sounds just to add some olives or fresh vegetables to your diet if your circumstances do not allow it. It is true that millions of people are regularly consuming the Sirtfoods discussed above, but significant numbers of people in the UK are not and the next chapter will attempt to provide an overview as to why this is the case.

Chapter 3: Calorie Restriction and Sirtuin Activation

"A long healthy life is no accident. It begins with good genes, but it also depends on good habits" Dan Buettner (explorer and endurance athlete)

Calorific Restriction (CR) as a mechanism by which to improve metabolism as part of what we would now term a balanced Plant based or Mediterr-Asian diet, is not a new undertaking. In terms of improved lifespan and quality of life the possible benefits of CR have been known since the 1930's. However, the idea that the SIRT proteins could improve these effects was established at around the year 2000. As such there is a long way to go before any definite assertions can be made. What can be said is that in laboratory animals different sirtuins have different effects on the physiology of the animals. From here it is fair to say that the potential for metabolic benefits derived from Sirtuin Activation (SA) could be augmented under conditions of a regulated CR diet. As of 2015 human trials have not been carried out and many of the experiments undertaken in the laboratory have been with genetically engineered animals. In other words these experiments were not carried out it in "real world" and are at this stage indicators of a potential (but likely) positive metabolic impact. Aside from these points the point is that the SIRT proteins can have enhanced metabolic impacts and will likely have long term benefits for the physiology and metabolism of mammals including human beings. Furthermore as has been made abundantly clear in this book a balanced and varied diet is a sure fire way to ingest the entirety of sirtuin activating chemicals. Hence once again there is no reason not to expand your diet irrespective of the writing presented below.

Specific chemicals present in the Mediterr-Asian diet such as resveratrol derived from red wine or oleuropein and hydroxytyrosol from olive oil and isoflavones from soybeans and ECGC are known to activate SIR1 proteins. Given the suggested roles of SIR1 in human metabolism some food scientists suggest that CR may increase this particular mode of action. From this position it is not unrealistic to infer that as part of a balanced diet and / or modulated dietary regimen that calorie restriction may boost the activation of all seven sirtuin proteins. One strand in the area of CR and SA concerns the hypothesised inhibition of serious health conditions such as Coronary Heart Disease CHD and Cardio Vascular Disease (CVD), type 2 diabetes, neurological disease as well as some forms of cancer. Additionally and irrespective of the actual mechanisms at work it appears that CR and the eating of polyphenol containing foodstuffs could have similar metabolic impacts on human beings. Furthermore a principle mechanism by which food derived polyphenols have their function amplified is through SA biochemistry. CR refers to a strict dietary protocol where the diet is reduced by any quantity up to 40%. When applied to micro-organism such as yeast, the glucose was cut by 40%, the budding lifespan of the yeast was significantly extended. It is not surprising that experimental findings such as these encourage interest in CR both as a method of extending quality and length of life in mammals. Research continues apace and findings continue to be contradictory, reflecting the complexity of the science being undertaken. For example, some studies suggest that the presence of yeast SIR2 is responsible for the increase in budding lifespan, others that its presence has no effect on reproduction. CR is a regimen that will have different impacts on different organs and therefore the entire human organism and these effects will vary between individuals. Hence there is no one size fits all approach and CR itself remains a deeply emotive area of research. As will be stressed again toward the end of this chapter it should only be carried out under the guidance of health care professionals. For our purposes there is a very real possibility that the activity of the sirtuins themselves may be augmented under the metabolic conditions induced by a CR regimen. In other words as the BMI (Body Mass Index) is reduced under the auspices of a Mediterr-Asian or Plant Based Diet (PBD) the very real benefits of Sirt Protein biochemistry are augmented.

The essential basis of CR is that it reduces levels of undesirable fats and LDL cholesterol (amongst other substances) in the blood stream as well as keeping the blood pressure within optimal homeostatic limits. All of these variables are implicated in both Coronary Heart Disease (CHD) and Cardio Vascular Disease (CVD). Furthermore the hormones leptin as indicated in chapter five and adiponectin in chapter 6 are key indicators of metabolic imbalance as expressed by their interaction with the hypothalamus. As numbers of adipose (fat) cells are steadily reduced leptin levels are reduced whilst those of adiponectin are increased and the appetite becomes balanced such that the person experiences the feeling of being "full" after they have eaten less food. Furthermore because adiponectin expresses anti-inflammatory, anti-atherogenic, insulin activity properties, it is highly likely to be protective against CVD and help with the treatment of type-2 diabetes.

Chapter two introduced the term "oxidative stress" and as we age our cells become more susceptible to its ravages. As biological molecules and organelles age they repair less readily and begin to accumulate in the cellular environment. Concurrently, the anti-oxidant capabilities of the body progressively degrade as we get older. In addition a perfect biologically negative storm arises as our metabolism changes because the production of ROS is widely to considered to increase in our later years. It is important to reiterate that the creation of ROS is a normal part of healthy metabolism and that the charged particles are not some sort of metabolic bogey man. At low concentrations ROS are known to benefit cellular processes in addition because the ROS cause a response at a molecular level in mammals (including ourselves) they induce adaptive effects which may well lead to new evolutionary pathways. As a whole ROS substances may garner long term benefit by acting as signalling molecules which could regulate the REDOX processes outlined in chapter 6. A managed program of CR could enhance such processes because when the body is not receiving new inputs of the metabolites of carbohydrate and fat digestion, more ROS species are produced when energy reserves are broken down.

SIRT 1 is often viewed as the gate keeper sirtuin against molecular and cellular oxidative stress as well as a protector against damage to nucleic acids, including DNA. During experiments on cell cultures researchers have demonstrated that during conditions of simulated CR that mammalian SIR1 activity is enhanced in the muscles, brain, kidneys and in adipose cells. The result as demonstrated by the experiments is that under conditions of CR numbers of adipose cells progressively decrease and as this occurs the body becomes more sensitive to the action of insulin. Intertwined with such a notion is research which suggests that under these circumstances SIRT 1 also promotes the action of those genes which promote glucose formation in the liver as opposed to that of glycogen. Simultaneously, SIRT 1 promotes the breakdown of fatty acids in the cell mitochondria. In the pancreas of laboratory animals the activation of SIRT 1 under conditions of CR promotes the increase of insulin and therefore breaks up of glycogen and fatty acids into glucose. At the same time the SIRT proteins in general are believed to protect the liver and other organs against the oxidative stress produced by changes in metabolism.

Having said all of this there is contradictory data concerning all of these suppositions such that there is equally robust research which suggests that under conditions of CR that the activity of all sirt proteins can be suppressed and may even elicit the opposite metabolic effects, such that fat is more readily synthesised and accumulated. However, these findings tend to be the result of feeding laboratory animals the equivalent of a human western diet. To further complicate matters different species of rodents expressed varying degrees of metabolic change. However, some of the discrepancy can be explained by diet such that the more fat (in particular saturated fat) the less effective where the SIRT proteins in general and SIRT 1 in particular. From this it is tentatively possible to suggest that a low fat diet promotes sirtuin activity and that for this activity to be most effective the diet itself must be balanced. In other words for the sirtuins to be effective the person must have balanced metabolism as indicated by an appropriate BMI. By definition a principle reason for embarking on any kind of CR is to lose weight and reduce the harm that a western diet causes to the circulatory system in particular and the rest of the body in general. Cardiovascular disease (CVD) is a huge killer and is characterised by high levels of LDL cholesterol, hardened and plaqued arteries (arthrosclerosis). Unsurprisingly in countries where the Western diet is the general norm CVD is a huge killer. According to the WHO CVD is the biggest cause of death across the world, accounting for over 30% of global mortality in 2012. During a regimen of CR SIR1 has been shown to inhibit inflammation and has been associated with decreased levels of both adipose tissue and cholesterol. Furthermore under these conditions the ability of the human body to excrete cholesterol and fat appear to be enhanced.

It is well understood that a degree of exercise is essential for healthy metabolism. In the human body there are various enzymes which are widely believed to activate the 7 sirtuin proteins. Science has yet to establish the precise mode of action of these relationships but strong indicators exist that in times of high energy expenditure and low energy inputs that energy sensing enzymes and cell signalling molecules have mutually beneficial synergistic relationship. In other words the sirtuin proteins are more active because they have stimulated to do so when the body is "burning off" its reserves of energy (i.e. fat cells). The research literature further implies that such responses are a normal physiological response to an increase in demand for chemical energy (i.e. from respiration). In addition it appears that during times of CR and other mechanisms of achieving metabolic balance that the process of autogaphy discussed in chapter six is enhanced. SIR1 is by far the most studies of the sirtuin proteins but as chapter one makes clear it is not the only one (pun intended). For example the efficacy sirtuins 3 and 4 promoted during times of CR, this is crucial because SIR3 is expressed in the brain, liver and kidneys and in a specific type of adipose tissue known as brown fat cells. One function of these cells is to act as an energy source in new born infants with the express purpose of generating the heat needed to maintain the body temperature at 37°C. As SIR3 is expressed that is brown fat cells are metabolised more rapidly, the activity of SIR4 is inhibited. This inhibition by series of exceptionally complex biochemical pathways (that we are far from fully understanding) stimulates the production of insulin and so could have utility in the treatment of diabetes.

All of this should give the reader the impression that the active compounds that are derived from a Mediterr-Asian and PBD do not act in isolation from each other. There are clear and definite relationships between these substances which collectively have a role in keeping the metabolism in balance and therefore the person healthier for a longer a period of time. A CR should never be attempted off the cuff that is without the consent of a health professional. It is simply not possible to maintain a full CR diet for long periods of time without undergoing significant tissue and organ wastage as well as reductions in everything from libido to cognitive function. If advised and under a properly controlled dietary regimen which is rich in the Sirtfoods discussed throughout this book, then a preventative and potential reversing effect may express itself. However, this is by no means guaranteed and CR still remains a highly emotive and controversial subject.

In 2013 researchers at the University of Washington established a mechanism by which SIR1 operates in the brain under periods of CR. In this example the research team showed that CR enhanced the activity of SIR1 on the hypothalamus (see chapter four) promoting increased activity inside the bones and muscles (the musculoskeletal system). The research is based on findings from experiments carried out on laboratory animals that had been genetically engineered to over express SIR1 in certain organs. The animals where fed a normal rodent diet and those that expressed the SIR1 in the brain were found to have improved musculoskeletal function. In addition the sleep pattern of this cohort of animals was much more regular than their peers; furthermore, this was associated with better temperature regulation and much more regular rates of respiration. Overall this cohort of mice lived longer, was healthier and was much less likely to develop the disease, preventable or otherwise. It is crucially important to impart that such research does not suggest that CR and SIRT activation mean that animals live longer. The researchers in this study are quick to state that the onset of ageing is postponed but not its pace, such that ageing and the potential for developing age related diseases is delayed but not stopped. In other words one day you are still going to depart this mortal coil, no matter how healthy you are. You are mortal deal with it! Having said that, the scientist involved have identified the parts of the hypothalamus and the specific genes that activate this segment of SIR1 biochemistry. The increase in signalling facilitated by SIR1 in the hypothalamus could prove to have significant implications for the prevention and treatment of the diseases associated with ageing. Intertwined with such findings is the knowledge that in experiments on insects and other arthropods and even yeast, a direct and positive relationship between SIR2 and ageing is clear and apparent. In other words those organisms with SIR2 in their adipose cells lived longer than those which did not.

In short as the remainder of this book will impart there is years of research ahead for those scientists in the field of nutrition and sirtuin biochemistry. However, a very solid foundation exists which sets the scene for further strong indicators of a causative connection between SA and CR in particular as well as diet in general. Such that the more foods which are known to contain SA's are eaten the more likely that the Sirt proteins will be activated, function together synergistically and holistically, to the overall benefit of our physiology.

Chapter 4: Perspectives on Malnutrition

"The best doctors give the least medicine" Benjamin Franklin

It cannot be overstated that the nutritional benefits of consuming Sirtfoods will only present themselves if you are consuming a balanced diet. Any high school biology text book will impart that to be balanced a diet must provide all of the nutrients in the correct amounts which allow the human organism to carry out its seven life processes. Malnutrition is generally associated with a situation in which people are not consuming enough of any of the principle food groups. These groups in their entirety contain the carbohydrates, fats, proteins as well as the vitamins, minerals, water and dietary roughage necessary for healthy living. Malnutrition is generally associated with situations where the organism has no alternative but to first breakdown its reserves of glycogen and then fats. This metabolism provides the energy needed to keep the body functioning but does not replace nutrients. The only mechanism by which mammals including human beings can replenish their stock of nutrients is by eating. Thus, if our nutrient reserves are not replaced by feeding the body will start to break down tissues such as muscle to stay alive. We understand this occurrence as starvation and it currently affects according to the UN Food and Agricultural organisation (UNFAO) approximately 800 million people globally. Far from being curtailed such instances of malnutrition are now increasingly occurring in the more prosperous countries.

Until the onset of the crisis and austerity economics it would have been fair to state that in the Western world access to and the affordability of food was overall not an issue. Irrespective of your income or social class most of us could afford to consume a balanced diet. When one considers the reality of food banks in the UK alone, it is equally fair to state that the above pronouncement no longer holds true. According to the Trussel Trust (a charity which seeks to end food poverty in the UK) over 1 million people are given weekly emergency food parcels to prevent the malnutrition we generally associate with the Global South (i.e. majority world). The picture across continental Europe is equally stark. According to the European Federation of Food Banks (EFFB) across the European Union (EU) over 125 million people are experiencing some degree of food poverty. Even the more affluent European countries such as Norway have now set up food banks to feed people who can no longer afford to purchase enough to eat. At the time of writing Oslo has the dubious honour of being the location for the EFFB's 257th European food bank. Unfortunately, these numbers look set to increase. Such is the negative impacts of cuts on the overall health of any nation, with the poor and most vulnerable members of society suffering disproportionately. Across the Atlantic Ocean US based NGO "Hunger Notes", asserts that almost 15% of all U.S households are experiencing food poverty. Put simply food poverty is a situation where people have to make an invidious choice between eating or heating, or feeding their children but not themselves. As of 2015 the number of people experiencing food poverty in the UK continues to rise. However, overall in parts of the world where the so called "western diet" is the norm an opposite form of malnutrition occurs. Instead of starving malnourished people in the Western world tend to be overweight or obese. These populations do not generally experience Kwashiorkor (protein deficiency) but do have an increased incidence of Type 2 diabetes, cardiovascular disease (stroke, heart attack, and atherosclerosis) as well as disorders of the skeletal system and even some forms of cancer. The consequences of the availability of cheap processed food which is high in fat, refined sugar and salt, whilst simultaneously being low in fibre, vitamins and minerals are clear and present. According to the WORLD HEALTH ORGANISATION a minimum of 2.8 million people are killed globally every year because of complications resulting from obesity. In the UK the figure is approximately 6% of the overall death rate which translates very roughly into several thousand deaths per year as of 2014. In short you can rest assured that if a population is not consuming its recommended 5 a day, then it certainly isn't getting its daily quota of Sirtfoods. Again it must be stressed, that Sirtfoods are not some wonder superfood; they are essential components of a balanced diet. As such they should be made available to all under the auspices of initiatives such as the Food for Life Partnership (FFLP).

It is undeniable that the global population is experiencing a profound obesity problem. Or more precisely the countries whose populations consume *"the western diet"* are experiencing a profound obesity problem. The word "obesity" is deceptively simple and the study of its causes and consequences spans across the major disciplines of the social, biological and chemical sciences. Thus, to answer the question *"what causes obesity?"* requires a holistic and considered response. At its most basic level obesity is a result of a convergence of the availability and consumption of foods which are processed and nutrient deficient in combination with a lack of regular exercise. Things become more complex when the relative availability and perceived affordability of so called *"junk food"* are compared to that of *"real food"*. A key thrust of this book is to state that integrating Sirtfoods (most of which already have established healthy eating benefits), should not be an issue provided you have access to them and can afford to buy them. Sadly, in modern Britain access to fresh wholesome and healthy food has become an issue for many communities. For instance, consider the reality of food deserts, a term which has entered popular parlance over the twenty years from 1995 to the present day. In the proverbial nutshell most people are aware of the health benefits of fresh fruit and vegetables. However, what happens if the community contains no outlets for any of the foods that are considered to be healthy or even worse people simply cannot afford to buy it. In such a context the nearest frozen food retailer or take away shop is going to be a much more attractive and convenient option. A food desert is loosely defined as any region where no reliable and affordable outlet for fresh fruit and vegetables exists within a set distance (anywhere up to 1000m) from a given residential community.

As of 2015 the number of food deserts in the UK is thought to several dozens and their existence is directly associated with dietary issues which fall under the term obesity. It is beyond the scope of this book to examine the causes of the wholly undesirable food desert phenomenon but their prevalence is correlated with the development of out of town supermarkets and the cutting back of essential public services, such as transport. Additionally, the phenomenon is not limited to the UK and it is not just a question of access. It is also a question of affordability and education. Over the years I've spoken to many of the younger generation who cannot tell the difference between different fruits and vegetables and many who have never opened up a cook book before or who even have a regular home prepared meal. In addition many of these children have answered *"from the supermarket"* when asked the question *"where does our food come from?"* These were not quintessentially deprived inner city children who had never seen a tree outside of a park before, but privileged European students in fee paying schools. I can categorically state that a lack of education around food does not respect social class. Additionally, I remember being taught at school and at home how to boil an egg or how to make different sauces. In my last year of secondary school we had "*survival cookery*" classes' last thing on Friday afternoons. I learnt how to make pasta, rice, pizza bases, bread and burgers (from scratch) as well dishes such as risotto. To my knowledge there is no commitment to any school (due to a lack of funding as opposed to intent) to offer home economics or domestic science (cooking) classes to their students. Without a doubt this and other factors concerning our "*connection to the food eat*" are contributors to the current dire situation.

As the 21st century progresses the number of obesity related deaths all over the Western world continues its annual increase. According to the World Health Organisation (WHO) obesity across the board has doubled over the 35 years since 1980. The figures speak for themselves; in 1980 approximately 800 million people were diagnosed as being clinically obese. At the time of writing the WHO estimates that approximately one third of the entire population (two billion people) are overweight and that 10% are clinically obese. Furthermore, a staggering 42 million children under 5 can now be categorised as overweight or obese. To make matters worse the numbers are actually increasing, such that by 2030 predictions of billions of people being obese (as opposed to merely being overweight) are not unusual. The truly shocking fact is that over half of this number lives in just 10 countries. The UK is likely to join this wholly undesirable club in a few short years. According to research published in the UK as of 2014, over half of the women and close two thirds of men are overweight or obese. Furthermore, suggestions that half of the population of the UK will be obese by 2050 are not unrealistic assertions.

The next chapter will look at how Sirtfoods can mitigate this form of malnutrition.

Chapter 5: Why are Sirtfoods so Beneficial?

"The doctor of the future will no longer treat the human frame with drugs, but rather will cure and prevent disease with nutrition." Thomas Edison

It suffices to impart that being "overweight" and being "obese" are different extremes of the same eating disorder. Irrespective of the cause obesity occurs when you consume more food and calories than your body needs to fulfill its energetic and life processing requirements. Any excess food is converted to fat which is then stored subcutaneously in the legs and abdomen. In other words obesity is a consequence of feeding more than metabolising. The fat in an obese person has accumulated to such an extent that healthy living and normal metabolic function is impaired. It is absolutely beyond the remit of this writing to explore in any great detail the social consequences of the sorry state of affairs outlined in the previous chapter. However, it is possible to extract several key factors and intimate how implementing a Sirtfood and balanced diet can reduce the social and economic consequences which are inextricably bound up in terms such as *"global obesity epidemic"*.

The most familiar method by which we define the terms overweight and obese is by use of a simple mathematical function we know as the Body Mass Index (BMI). Whilst there are several issues with the methodology concerning BMI calculations, the health impacts of being obese are clear and present.

The calculation is very simple:

Body Mass in Kg / Height in Metres = BMI

The World Health Organisation (WHO) defines an obese person as having a BMI of more than 30 and you are overweight if your BMI exceeds 25. In extreme cases a BMI of over 40 delimits, chronic and potentially life threatening severe obesity. The numerical outcome of this simple equation is used to establish a base line from which to ascertain the broad strokes concerning an individual's eating habits. In other words the BMI is not a diagnosis of obesity it is an indicator. However, to be distracted by this fact is to take the next left turn to the confused town known as semantics, the economic alone cost is staggering. For example research published by the McKinsey Global Institute (a global management consultancy) in November 2014 outlines the reasons why obesity costs the UK economy some £47 Billion per year, which translates to a loss of 3% in GDP. Globally the MGI report states that obesity constitutes 5% of the global death rate and a loss of approximately $2 trillion, which is about 3% of GDP.

The social cost to the UK in terms of NHS treatment for conditions such as stroke, type 2 diabetes, Cardiovascular conditions, breast and colon cancer as well as a whole host of other ailments is calculated to be about £6 billion per year, currently the UK spends around 1% on obesity prevention programmes. On top of this huge figure an additional £10 billion is spent on treatment for diabetes related to obesity. In other words £16 billion is spent annually on treating conditions that are by and largely preventable. To put things into perspective the total financial commitment to dealing with obesity is more than is spent on the police, probation, law courts and fire brigade, combined. The MGI report suggests that if nothing is done then by 2030 the figure for treating obesity (excluding type 2 diabetes) alone could balloon to £12 billion; by any benchmark this is clearly unacceptable. Overall, the MGI report recommends a coordinated response to the problem; such a response includes nutritional education and provision of healthy school and work place meals, which are affordable for all, the parallels with FFLP should be obvious. It advocates a school curriculum which integrates exercise and domestic science. It sees the benefits of the provision of facilities ranging from more cycle lanes to subsidised membership for gyms and health clubs. The report contains many other excellent suggestions and solutions which are aimed at individuals and communities, but also says that funding for such initiatives is essential. All of these initiatives have the capacity to help and to quote the director of the MGI *"Efforts to address obesity have been piecemeal up till now. Yet obesity is a systemic issue, born of many interlocking factors, and only a systemic response will do."* I could not have put it better myself, except to add that there is no magic bullet or wand waving based solution.

Obesity is an example of a non-communicable disease, which means it cannot be spread by the same mechanisms by which infectious diseases are spread. The condition is for most of us an acquired characteristic meaning that if you are avoiding (or at least limiting) processed foods then you are unlikely to become obese. Having stated that, there is a large body of research which infers a genetic basis for obesity, which will not be discussed here. Suffice to say in this frame, the requirements of the body have been met but the hypothalamus does not respond to the action of hormones such as leptin and consequently the person takes longer to experience the sensation of feeling full. It is completely fair to state that there is a strong element of individual and community responsibility for obesity, but as the previous chapter sets out this is only part of the explanation. The simplest and most obvious mechanism by which to obviate the obesity epidemic is to shape food choices by ensuring that healthy eating options are affordable, accessible and readily available. In other words the elimination of food deserts and providing facilities by which people can exercise regularly and within their budget, all of this of course requires investment. Unfortunately, in the UK such funding is woefully lacking, for instance the FFLP partnership mentioned in Chapter 3 is almost totally dependent on funding from the national lottery, in my view this is akin to using a sticking plaster to treat a gangrenous wound. The FFLP is the proven mechanism by which to improve the diet of millions of children and should be rolled nationally as a matter of priority. It is these sorts of initiatives that will enable the recommendations of agencies such as the MGI to translate into the necessary level of action. Intertwined with such a position is the role of the food industry and their bedfellows, the supermarkets. One could write an encyclopaedia on this relationship but one of its consequences is the fact that as of 2014 UK citizens are spending billions of pounds every year on ready meals. Some of his expenditure is in response to the on-going recession, whereby so called *"high end lines"* or *"supermarket take away boxes"* are substituting eating out. However, the fact remains that the UK ranks top of the ready meal consumption league, at least as far as Europe is concerned. Overall the UK has the worst obesity statistics in Europe, but only just. The bottom line is that the food industry must share the responsibility for the obesity problem alluded to in the previous chapters, to suggest otherwise is a cognitive dissonance bordering on denial. Put simply, the manufacturers should be compelled to move away from processed foods such as ready meals which are generally loaded with fat, sugar, salt and more individual additives and *"E"* numbers than there are characters on my key board. Furthermore there should be a massive program of diverting resources toward making healthy eating choices available at the expense of processed foods. The industry as a whole should be regulated such that, as one positive development, it is illegal to advertise junk food to children and teenagers. Such regulations ought to apply to the global junk food outlets. Again, this is not an exhaustive list it is only a scratch on the surface, but if obesity is to be genuinely treated as the new smoking then these are exactly the kind of initiatives which need to be pushed forward with the utmost urgency. According to the MGI report a reduction of obesity levels to 1993 levels will eliminate 5 million cases of obesity related disease and save the NHS at least £1 Billion annually. To put it alternatively the totality of interventions suggested in the MGI report could (according to its researchers) bring a fifth of obese and overweight people to a BMI which is less than 25. To my mind this is an absolute minimum. OK so there we have the big picture to coin the phrase *"what can you and I do, right now immediately, forthwith and with great gusto?"*

In my view the simplest way to integrate Sirtfoods into your diet is to go through the recipes in your favourite cook book. What's that you say, *"You don't have a cook book"*, well, if you don't have a good cook book then you are in remiss, so you must get hold of one. I mean for sure there are thousands of recipes on line and dozens of exceptionally talented chefs with equally honed communication skills to help you cook them. That is all well and good, but a decent cookbook is absolutely essential for any kitchen. Speaking personally I am not a fan of what is called *"nouveau cuisine"* and I simply cannot abide restaurants that are all style and no substance. Think large plates with equally large prices but oppositely sized servings and you'll see where I am coming from. In short I see it as pretentious nonsense and equally the inverse of proper wholesome food. Ok that's that sorted! So what type of cook book should you get? Well there really is no set answer and you certainly don't need a brand new one. I got the two I use the most from a charity shop; others were picked up at the local car boot sale. Speaking personally I come from the no nonsense step by step explanation of how to make everything from decent omelettes or full (variation in a theme) English breakfasts to gourmet meals that are designed to impress. Step forward roasted guinea fowl with pomegranate and braised greens (kale and spinach) with roasted vegetables, or for a 90% vegan like myself, all the above minus the Guinea Fowl.

My favourite style of cook book is the traditional farmhouse type or those of the Delia Smith variety. The reason is simple there are sections on how to make and prepare every dish you can conceivably think of. In fact such books are a mine of information and contain all the advice you could possibly need plus the necessary nutritional advice as well as the definite no-nos. In this world of celebrity chefs I love the no-nonsense style of Nigel Slater and Gordon Ramsey (although the expletives are not always necessary, but hey that's marketing for you!). I have to say I have a healthy respect for Jamie Oliver, simply because the man can cook and constantly talks about "connecting with food", but more so for his tireless work to bring healthy foods to the schools and general public. A further piece of advice is to get your proverbial pantry filled with some staple ingredients that is herbs, spices, pulses, as well as various seasonings and flavourings. Many of which add to your SA's by default!

There is no great mystery to cooking, cheffing up, getting something together and most definitely quick and fast does not mean junk food. Put simply, if you can read a book and operate a cooker then you are able to eat healthily; even if some meals are somewhat unorthodox! For example consider the omelette my girlfriend has just made, a loose interpretation of a 30 year old Delia Smith recipe. Another reason why I love the more traditional and basic looking books, is to state that *"if it's not broken, it doesn't need fixing"*. The Sirtfood contingent is composed of olives and onions whilst the eggs bind together mushrooms tomatoes, one roast potato, a slice of stuffing, a smidgen of grated cheddar and some baked beans. All of it gently fried in a very thin layer of olive oil. Yes it's left over surprise, but it contains ALL the food groups and took 10 minutes to make. In addition, the moral aspects are satisfied, after all we live in a world were about 1Billion people are going without enough to eat, thus it is totally unacceptable to throw food away. So when you are cooking do not be stingy, but don't overdo it either and any excess should be portioned up for those times when you are in a hurry.

OK, back to the omelette! I am now fully energised and nutritionally stocked up until tea time when we will be having a Sirt food laden meal (courtesy of kale) tomato sauce with pasta. The great thing about making any sauce is that as long as you get the proportions about right you can make as much as you like. So you can make a shed load and then freeze what you don't use for another time. At this point it's worth pointing out that you could do with having some frozen stocks in your freezer. Believe me, freezing any surplus or intentionally making more than you need does save you time in the long run.

Chapter 6: SIRT proteins, Activation and Processes Affected

"Today, more than 95% of all chronic disease is caused by food choice, toxic food ingredients, nutritional deficiencies and lack of physical exercise." Mike Adams (The Health Ranger and Natural News editor)

Metabolism is a complex series of inter-related biological processes which work collectively to maintain homoeostasis. In biology homoeostasis refers to maintaining every conceivable metabolic or biological process you can think of, irrespective of external conditions, within optimal conditions. For example your body temperature is not maintained at 37°C because it's a nice integer. The dissipation of the heat released as glucose is oxidised in the mitochondria and is regulated to maintain a body temperature of 37°C. This temperature is the optimum for the thousands of enzymes, including the SIRT enzymes which are so crucial to our metabolism. If this temperature is not maintained due to conditions such as hyperthermia (heat exhaustion), then many enzymes are said to denature. In one sentence this means that they lose the ability to catalyse metabolic reactions and so the processes that keep us alive begin to slow down or in extreme cases can actually stop altogether. Other variables such as acidity (pH levels) govern the efficiency of enzymes. For instance, salivary amylase will function in the near neutral (pH 6.2-7.4) conditions of the mouth. However, it would denature completely in the stomach where the protease enzymes are designed to work in the extremely acidic conditions of the stomach. An additional example concerns the role of anti-oxidants, and yes we are returning to this notion of a balanced diet. If too many anti-oxidants are consumed through feeding (or more likely they are ingested in supplement form), then the immune system can become compromised. Put simply the immune system requires minimum levels of free radicals (which will be discussed below), in the lymphatic and circulatory systems. In a related frame there is research from Scandinavia which asserts that excessive concentrations of anti-oxidants, actually promotes the growth of certain tumours, at least in laboratory animals. Furthermore, and perhaps to demonstrate the point that eating healthily beats supplements hands down, other research indicates that too much resveratrol may nullify the proven benefits of regular exercise. These studies concerned excessively high doses of resveratrol which are far in excess of those one could expect from normal eating habits. This chapter will hopefully inculcate that compounds such as resveratrol are likely to have multiple roles in a properly functioning metabolism. Hence the reader is once again asked to sear that word balance and its slightly nerdy cousin homeostasis into their consciousness.

Resveratrol is thought to induce the production of a substance called endothelial nitric oxide, which stimulates the dilation of blood vessels. An endothelium is any layer of cells which covers any organ, but is most associated with vessels of the lymphatic and circulatory system. Hence resveratrol may have a role in maintaining an optimum body temperature during periods of exercise and exposure to high ambient temperatures. From this position research has indicated that resveratrol may play a part in alleviating hypertension. Other studies considered the role of supplements as opposed to consuming Sirtfoods properly. That is consumed as they were meant to be eaten, in leaf or berry form and not as dietary supplement pill. It has (I hope) been well established that diet is preferable to supplements and that field of SIRT protein research could lead to quantifiable benefits in terms of reducing obesity (malnutrition) in the industrialised world. We have established that eating Sirtfoods as part of a future and state run healthy eating programme would result in a massive reduction in obesity levels. However this statement does not explain the biochemical mechanisms which need to be functioning properly to achieve it. In other words it is self-evident that calorific restriction and ditching the junk and processed food will get your BMI down to the correct level, but how does this occur in biochemical terms?

Well first we need to explain what is meant by calorific restriction (CR), it's important because all of the processes outlined below are much more effective if the person is restricting their intake of unhealthy foods. OK here we go, CR as the term suggests is a mechanism by which it is possible to ingest all of your nutritional requirements without piling on the calories. In dietary terms a calorie is a unit employed to measure the energy content (as opposed to nutritional content) of a given food. All circumstances being equal the more calories that you ingest the more chance you have of becoming overweight or obese and/ or the more exercise you need to partake in. As we saw in the opening chapters the Sirtfoods are a range of high nutrient low energy foods. It must also be said that the more plant based matter that is eaten as compared with meat and to a lesser extent fish, the fewer calories you will ingest. In the context of obesity one does not need a PhD to assert that removing saturated fats will very quickly reduce your calorie intake. Research in the field of CR stretches back to the early years of the 20th century, but it is only in the last few years that mechanisms have been established which explain how it may work in the body. Overall, under the instruction of health professional CR will have benefits to a person provided it does not lead to malnutrition. In particular it has been shown to promote longevity and one mechanism by which this is thought to occur is through a process known as autophagy.

As stated in chapter one, living cells are the building blocks from which all organisms are made. As with all means of construction, the tools will eventually wear out and the same is true of cells and their components (the organelles). For instance red blood cells are manufactured in the bone marrow to replace those that are worn out and transported to the liver and spleen, where they are broken down. Every day approximately 2 million red blood cells are removed and replaced without compromising the ability of the blood stream to fulfil its transport function. The same is true of sub-cellular processes and the organelles which make them possible. In autophagy damaged or worn organelles are removed and replaced and the scientific literature imparts that SIRT1 has significance for the autophagy of mitochondria. From here it can be inferred that other SIRT proteins are involved in the autophagy of other organelles and that the homeostatic balance between removal of old organelles and the creation of new structures is an essential component of healthy metabolism. Such inferences have yet to be formally demonstrated but a role for the SIRT proteins is considered to be a possibility. However, a word of caution must be expressed to the reader.

Any assertion that a substance will increase the lifespan of any organism is sure to raise a few eyebrows and be greeted with a degree of popular and scientific scepticism. I mean let's be honest, the life extending properties of one substance or another have been extolled by different human cultures for thousands of years. It is well understood that in the ancient world the deities worshipped were seen as immortal by the mere puny mortals that worshipped them. In most of these cultures the source of immortality was normally connected to some form of food or infusion (elixir) that only the deity concerned was allowed to consume. A cursory look through the mythology of the ancient world makes reference to substances such as ambrosia or noma which could be consumed to extend the life of the mortals (that is people). Accordingly, the notion that SRT1 could extend the life of the common fruit fly (the Drosophila species so beloved of biological research) and certain nematodes, let alone human beings, has rightly been greeted with a healthy dose of solid scientific doubt. However, ever since the discovery in 2012 that SIRT6 could increase longevity in mice by 15%, interest in this aspect of sirtuin biology has far from waned. Evidence for longevity comes from a 2006 study which showed that mice that had been genetically engineered to be deficient in SIRT6 displayed the characteristics of ageing much more rapidly than their peers. The compound SIRT6 is believed to have a role in repairing cellular DNA and the transgenic mice that were lacking in this protein had all died within a month. When one considers that the life span of the average mouse is about a year, the implications are obvious. However, it cannot be stated that any of the sirtuin proteins is directly involved in prolonging the life of any mammalian species.

Additionally, the SIRT proteins do not operate in isolation from each other and as such they are likely to be involved in different biochemical processes. It is also not outside the bounds of possibility to state that the different modes of action are likely to have synergistic benefits to the organism. For instance in the above research the transgenic mice had been genetically engineered to develop malignant tumours. Concurrently, SIRT6 is widely believed to have a role in preventing certain cancers so if a mouse is deficient in that particular protein then the likelihood of developing tumours will increase. In other words there is no direct causative evidence that SIRT 6 or indeed the other Sirt promote longevity per se. What can be said with a high degree of confidence is that the Sirt proteins in general and SIRT6 in particular could affect the incidence of the biological characteristics of ageing. In addition, there is more than anecdotal evidence that the conditions associated with the ageing of the SIRT6 deficient mice could have been down to the consequences of excessively low and chronically depressed blood sugar levels. A further factor is gender. Irrespective of any research concerning Sirt proteins in mice, female mice live longer than male mice. In male mice that have been engineered to over express SIRT6 the animals simply caught up with the females who were the control or placebo group. In this frame it is important to remember that with homo-sapiens and many other mammals, there are good sound biological and evolutionary reasons as to why females live longer than males. Sorry guys (including yours truly) but the chances are that a far as longevity is concerned it will be a *"beast behind the door"* scenario, written by the internationally acclaimed author *"Hugo First"*.

In Secondary school one of the first metabolic processes that students learn about is aerobic respiration. Hence it seems appropriate to explore how calorific restriction and Sirtfoods could well benefit this most fundamental metabolic process. Glucose is the simplest carbohydrate and is the principle source of energy in living cells. The aerobic (oxygen present) respiration which occurs in every cell of our bodies is in effect a combustion reaction. In the mitochondria a complex series of reactions converts glucose to carbon dioxide and water and provide the energy needed for metabolism. Often the mitochondria are referred to as the power house of a healthy cell. For every mole (chemical counting unit) of glucose that is oxidised (reacted in the presence of oxygen) approximately

2830KJ (686 kilo calories) of energy is released. This works out to be approximately 4 calories per gram of glucose. In chemical reactions energy is obtained via the breaking of chemical bonds. The energy is not created it is transferred from the glucose molecules to an intermediary known as Adenosine Tri-Phosphate (ATP) which then transfers the energy through the cell. Often ATP will be referred to as the energy currency of living cells. There is a hefty amount of research which holds that SIRTSs 3-5 may finely tune the rate of respiration such that it occurs in line with the rate of nutrient (glucose) supply. In addition to ATP transfers chemical energy throughout the cell it is broken down, the only way it can be reused as the energy currency is if it is rebuilt back into ATP. This process is termed oxidative phosphorylation and is catalysed by SIRT 3. In addition SIRT 3 is thought to influence ketosis in the liver as well as the rate of ammonia removal during the breakdown of amino acids in the liver. Ketosis is the first stage of the fatty acid breakdown outlined below.

Further research in the activity of SIRT5 in this vital metabolic function continues apace. As stated above the SIRT proteins are likely to have a variety of functions and their activity can equally likely be triggered by different metabolic circumstances. For instance, if the body reduces its nutrient intake such that person is effectively fasting SIRT 1 protein has been shown to have a role in the function of the mitochondria in organs such as the liver and in the muscle fibres. The research literature is replete with indicators that the rate at which the cells construct mitochondria could be influenced by how energetic the cell is, that is the rate at which it is respiring. Overall, the supposition is that the presence of certain nutrients may act as a trigger to SIRT 1 (and to a lesser extent SIRT 3) and that in turn may increase the rate at which respiration occurs. In other words if you are following a Calorific Restriction / Sirtfood diet your cells are receiving more nutrients and glucose molecules and are functioning more efficiently. They are in effect operating within homeostatic limits. Metabolic diseases such as obesity are correlated with malfunctioning mitochondria. A further strand of research which may have implications for the treatment of diabetes is the presence (or not) of a hormone known as adiponectin, a protein and hormone that is only secreted from fat (adipose) cells. Adiponectin has a direct influence on the metabolism of fats and carbohydrates such as glucose. Its action has also been linked to the activity and presence of SIRT 1. Studies conducted on laboratory animals show that increasing levels of adiponectin in the general circulation provokes increased mitochondrial activity and by association the construction of mitochondria inside the cell. (Personally I do not support vivisection or any other type of animal experimentation but I feel I have to report the research and insights deduced). In addition because proteins are coded for by our DNA this relationship may well add extra weight to arguments concerning the genetic basis of obesity.

Related to the respiration of glucose is the metabolism of lipids (fats). In their entirety fats are an energy reserve which is stored as a layer of adipose (subcutaneous) tissue which is found on the lower end of the dermis (the skin) and has the dual function of acting as an insulating layer (fats are poor conductors of heat). A third function for fats in the body is to carry fat soluble vitamins to the cells of the body which use them. In other words fats are essential molecules, the trick is to modulate your intake and ingest the correct type that is the unsaturated variety. Fats are formed by two principle actions; first three soluble fatty acid molecules are chemically bonded to a substance known as glycerol. Hence fat molecules are often referred to as tri-glycerides. The second mechanism is through the action of insulin and that means we must very quickly revisit glucose. In the blood stream when glucose levels reach a high enough level the hypothalamus (part of the brain that controls homeostasis) sends a hormonal signal to the pancreas so that specialist cells known as *"beta"* cells secrete the hormone insulin. This stimulates all cells in the body to take up glucose and convert it to glycogen. This effect is most pronounced in the liver where the glycogen is stored until it is needed. The process that produces glycogen is known as glycolysis, thus glycogen is in effect thousands of individual glucose molecules attached to each other by what is termed a glycosidic bond. Hence, both glucose and glycogen are readily available energy sources whose relative concentrations are regulated by the action of the hormones insulin and glucagon. The latter hormone is released when glucose levels fall low enough for the hypothalamus to signal the *"alpha"* cells in the pancreas to release it. The release of glucagon stimulates the liver to convert the glycogen back into glucose (glucogenesis) by breaking the glycosidic bonds between each glucose molecule in the glycogen molecule. This another example of homeostasis and when the system breaks down type 2 diabetes can develop (Type 1 is ignored for the purpose of this writing). It is well established that Sirts-3-5 congregate around the mitochondria. Thus, it is fair to assert that Sirts3-5 are likely to have an essential role in regulating cellular respiration.

Once all cells in the body have enough glucose to meet their needs and the liver and muscles are packed with glycogen, glucose is converted to fatty acid and in turn chemically bonded to the glycerol molecule and then transported to the adipose layer. If a person is overweight or obese they do not necessarily have more fat cells than a person who is not. It is more that each fat cell contains more fat molecules. Once you have accumulated excess fat it is very difficult to remove unless you change your diet, principally, because fats are such a concentrated store of energy. It takes a lot of exercise before the body starts to break down fatty acids in aerobic respiration. Hence, the best course of action is prevention as opposed to cure! In very general terms the body will use its reserves of glucose and glycogen before it starts to break down fat reserves. A diet rich in Sirtfoods and plant matter in general contains more nutrients and fewer carbohydrates than the western diet outlined previously. Hence you are less likely to gain weight via the ingestion of nutritionally questionable foods. In extreme cases of obesity that may require surgery to remove excess fat a surgeon or doctor will likely prescribe a calorific restriction diet regime. This is simply because the body has to start burning off its stores of fat and won't do that whilst the person is still ingesting carbohydrates. Fats are much more concentrated store (as opposed to source) of energy. On average each mole of fat contains approximately 9 grams of energy and we have between 50 and 200 billion fat cells. Once your sugar levels are being properly maintained the body can start breaking down the fatty acids. SIRT3 is thought to have a function in the oxidation of fatty acids, which is the first stage of their breakdown. The trick is to get your body into a position to start the metabolism of fat cells. The first stage of which is the ketosis mentioned above.

If you are overweight or obese the only way you are going to burn off your excess fat is by avoiding foods which are high in refined sugar and fats. That is foods which are the total opposite of Sirtfoods and its more proscriptive variant the calorific restriction (C.R.) diet. Your body will use glucose and glycogen first and if you keep ingesting excessive carbohydrates (which are metabolised to sugars such as glucose) all you will succeed in doing is replenishing your reserves of glucose or worse actually increasing your BMI. You will need to follow a genuinely balanced diet in which fresh Sirtfoods will play a part. Or follow the instructions of a surgeon pertaining to a CR diet. Helpfully, SIRT1 and SIRT3 have been shown to have a function in detecting the presence of the products of digestion. These products are in effect the nutrients the body needs and their presence (or not) influences the activity of other proteins inside the mitochondria. Perhaps to underline the point about balance, in instances of caloric restriction (i.e. fasting), SIRT 3 in effect goes into overdrive. The protein will activate and then inhibit the action of a whole range of enzymes and protein function in general and in this context SIRT 3 has been associated with modulating conditions ranging from the cardiovascular to diabetes and hearing loss.

SIRT1 is found in many mammals and is most active when feeding is problematic for the organism. It is equally active when a calorific restriction (CR) diet is imposed. It also has a fundamental role in the biology of free radical clean-up which is discussed below. It is also considered to have a profound role in regulating the cell cycle and therefore cellular lifespan. This assertion clearly has implications for the treatment of cancer and stress related conditions. As a regulator of metabolism and respiration it is known to accelerate the rate at which cells aerobically convert glucose to its metabolites (CO_2 and H_2O). Furthermore SIRT1 has been shown to suppress the storage of fats whilst simultaneously increasing the rate of processes such as ketosis. Thus SIRT1 can potentially reduce the incidence of conditions ranging from heart attacks to osteoporosis, in short the conditions associated with both obesity and old age. It must be restated that science is a long way from demonstrating the exact mechanisms by which all the SIRT compounds garner their metabolic benefits, but the research is continuing. Overall good diet raises the levels of SIRT 1 and there is no reason to suppose that the same effect can be produced with the other 6 SIRT compounds.

Any discussion of SIRT proteins would be incomplete without some mention of substances known as free radicals. In what is perhaps one of the great ironies of life on planet Earth, the production of certain types (species) of charged atoms of oxygen are known to have a damaging effect on the biological molecules which are essential for cell integrity and function. Other species of atom such as hydrogen and nitrogen are also known to exert similar effects which fall under the term "*Cellular Oxidative Stress*" (COS). It is molecules referred to as free radicals that are thought to promote COS, so we must ask how this works. Electrons are the sub-atomic and negatively charged particles which occupy the empty space around the nucleus. When an atom is electrochemically balanced the number of positively charged protons (in the nucleus) will equal the number of electrons which spin around the nucleus in electron clouds. Electrons themselves are most stable when they exist together in pairs. A free radical forms in atoms when the electron pairs are split and the particles are separated from each other. Such separation of electron pairs is a common feature of many biological processes. A free radical is a highly energetic form of an atomic substance and for our purposes we are most interested in oxygen. In a free radical state the species of atom is seeking to off load its surplus of energy and in the firing line are biological molecules ranging from fats to Deoxy-Ribonucleic Acid (DNA). The phrase "*COS*" is a catch all term used to describe damage caused by reactive oxygen species (ROS). In other words any molecule which carries at least one unpaired electron can cause damage to biological molecules inside living cells as well as those which exist on its membrane. However, there is no need to panic! It all comes back to the phrase *"balanced diet"*. Provided the diet contains an abundance of anti-oxidants, the impact of the free radicals is curtailed.

In their entirety the SIRT enzymes are widely believed to protect cells from the attentions of free radical molecules which love nothing better than to pass on their excess energy to any takers. They in effect promote the activity of other biological molecules (not limited to enzymes), such that excess free radicals are chemically reduced. You may recall from secondary (high) school chemistry the mnemonic (OILRIG). The initials refer to the movement of electrons and they mean oxidation is loss and reduction are a gain of electrons. In chemistry the reactivity of a substance is determined by the position and numbers of electrons which are furthest from the nucleus. Atomic theory shows us that the negatively charged electrons orbit the nucleus in orbital clouds and they are held in place by the protons of the nucleus, which have a positive charge. An atom is said to be electrochemically stable when the number of electrons and protons is equal. The electrons themselves are most stable when they orbit the nucleus in pairs. During the course of our metabolism it is perfectly normal for radical species such as reactive oxygen species (ROS) to be produced. Hence we have over millions of years evolved processes which effectively hoover up the free radicals which *"can"* (emphasis) cause damage to biological molecules in, on and around the cell. These species of atom are reactive because they have so much excess energy; the only way they can lose this energy is by chemically reacting with any substance that they come into contact with. When this happens the free radical is chemically reduced and the biological molecule is oxidised. Hence for chemical reactions which involve reduction and oxidation the term *"redox"* is applied and both processes occur simultaneously.

The compound which is oxidised loses its electrons to the substance it is reacting with; hence the second reacting substance is reduced. Now, to really confuse you! A substance which is termed a *"reducing agent"* is said to cause oxidation because the reducing agent causes the oxidised substance to lose electrons to the reducing agent. In other words the oxidised substance loses electrons and the reduced substance gains the *same* electrons. Conversely an "oxidising agent" is said to cause reduction because it loses electrons to a second reacting substance, which is itself reduced. Practically all chemical reactions fall under the term *"redox"* and if you're flummoxed don't worry. Please feel free to read this section again and follow up on the previous hyperlinks! For our purposes all you need to appreciate is that the free radical is the reducing agent and the biological molecules are the source of extra electrons. The Sirt proteins are believed to act themselves as either the electron source or more likely activate so called oxygen scavenging substances. For example SIRT 3 has been shown to activate enzymes which are prolific scavengers of reactive oxygen species (ROS). In other words the anti-oxidant reduces the free radicals it comes into contact while it is simultaneously oxidised. In so doing the free radical loses electrochemical energy to the anti-oxidant and not to essential biological molecules. This underpins a fundamental tenet of chemical reactivity. Namely, that substances react with each other to become more energetically stable and that as this stability is achieved, no new electrons are made, they are transferred or shared between reacting substances, forming new compounds in the process. Overall, the SIRT proteins appear to have a definite function in regulating COS *"Cellular Oxidative Stress"* and so may have an indirect effect in curtailing the development of degenerative disease and other less serious conditions that are associated with aging.

Stress is a highly subjective occurrence and is expressed differently in different people, irrespective of the circumstances. In biological terms stress occurs when the body responds in a physiological manner due to the result of a stimulus or sensory input. The stress response is highly beneficial to the survival of the organism; one must only look at the *"fight or flight"* response to seeing this assertion exemplified. In its entirety stress is an entirely predictable and normal biological occurrence which induces a change in behaviour which is designed to remove the organism from the stressing event or enable it to be accommodated. The physiological basis of the stress response is the action of the hormones Cortisol and noradrenalin which are secreted from the adrenal glands situated on the kidneys. The stress response signals the body that it has to prepare for either *"fighting"* or *"flighting"* or possibly both and is only beneficial while the event is occurring. A huge burst of energy fuelled by the aerobic respiration of glucose promotes the feeling of being alert and primed for action. This is a normal facet of our evolution and is absolutely essential to our survival. Consider what would happen if you did not respond quickly and rapidly to a fast moving vehicle that was coming right at you? The same question could be asked of the first humans as they sought to avoid predation.

Problems begin to develop when the feeling of being *"stressed"* is regular and / or constant. Consequently, the body does not have the opportunity to re-adjust back to a less stressed state. Stress hormone levels can reach very high levels in the blood stream which can present serious health risks not dissimilar to those associated with obesity. In other words chronic stress results in systemic changes to the biochemistry and metabolism of the stressed person. These changes announce their impact in the form of diseases or conditions including:

- Circulatory and pulmonary systems (heart, lungs and circulation)

- Obesity and related conditions such as diabetes

- Hypertension

- Immune system where the functioning of B and T cells is impaired

- Insomnia and associated depression and lethargy

- Osteoporosis and other physical conditions associated with ageing

- Dementia including but not limited to Alzheimer's disease

In terms of neurological impacts elevated and chronic levels of cortisol in the blood stream are viewed as dangerous because of the impact on the hippocampus (part of the brain which deals with memory and thought). Although no causative link has as yet been established the evidence suggests that the brains of highly stressed persons are smaller than those of their unstressed counterparts. The culprit being a reduced volume hippocampus which is implicated in the memory and cognitive deficits associated with dementia. It is important to underline that the stress response itself is not dangerous; however, being in a heightened state of stress as a result of a messy divorce, a workplace dispute or even the bi-daily rush hour can all trigger a long term stress response. The list of triggers is endless and will almost certainly be different for different people. To avoid the risks associated with elevated levels of stress hormones the body needs time to break them down into harmless substances which can either be re-assimilated or expelled. In what is known as the cortisol / adrenal switch the time taken for cortisol and nor-adrenaline to become toxins is limited. In other words the time taken for a substance to start behaving as a toxin has a major influence on how the body deals stressing events. If the body does not have time to cope with stressing events then the beneficial aspects of the stress response are morphed into a set of symptoms (such as those mentioned above) which can be catastrophic for the person.

In all human cells (aside from the gametes and red blood cells) there are 23 pairs of chromosomes. These are the structures which contain the molecules of DNA and on the end of each DNA molecule is a structure known as a telomere. The complete structure and function of telomeres are not fully understood but they have a vital role in keeping living cells biologically fit for purpose. With each cell division the telomeres become shorter and hence cells have a limited lifespan. One facet of the biology of a chronically stressed person is the extent to which their stress is expressed at a cellular level. The disappearance of telomeres causes a condition known as cellular senescence, where the cell is alive but no longer capable of reproduction. This process is widely believed to be the genetic basis for ageing. In people who are chronically stressed the action of the hormone cortisol interferes with the enzyme telomerase which catalysis the chemical reactions that repair telomeres. As an example of why the diet must be balanced it is recognised that excessive amounts of ECGC inhibit the action of telomerase and the processes which manufacture proteins in the ribosomes.

In certain species of yeast SIRT2 has been observed to help prolong the life of individual cells. Research shows us that SIRT2 is most present in the cell during asexual reproduction (mitosis) where they congregate around the chromosomes as they divide. To be precise the SIRT 2 proteins congregate around a single strand of DNA (a chromatid) which is found in the nucleus of the daughter cell immediately after it has separated from the parent cell. Clearly, this suggests a role for this protein in the successful reproduction of living cells. Thus if ageing is directly associated with a reduction in the length of telomeres and if SIRT2 is associated with dividing chromosomes and therefore the successful copying of genetic information, then a confluence of stress, SIRT activity and diet clearly presents itself. SIRT1 is widely believed to contribute to the free radical clean up outlined in the section on free radicals. Any substance which reduces the impact of "*Cellular Oxidative Stress*" must by definition contribute to the over health of the person (or other living organism). SIRT1 has been shown to catalyse the biochemical reactions which hoover up the free radical substances in the manner described above. In addition SIRT1 has been shown to have a role in maintaining an optimal telomere length and because it is known to contribute to what geneticists call gene silencing it could influence the onset of age related diseases that have a genetic basis. This is a convenient juncture at which to point out that when we are referring to the longevity benefits of Sirtuin Activators (SA's) we are talking about treating conditions associated with ageing. If this conditions can be treated such as through stem cell science then they may well contribute to a longer life span. You are still going to "age" in the truest sense of the word but it is entirely possible that the biological conditions we associate with old age may well become treatable.

At the same time SIRT2 may well have a role in ensuring that the enzymes which are responsible for copying DNA and synthesising new proteins function properly. Overall SIRT2 may have a role in regulating the success and rate of protein synthesis and the recombination of DNA during mitosis as well as ensuring that the sub-telomeric region of each DNA molecule is properly maintained. This is the region of each chromosome just next to each telomere and is thought to act as a buffer between the telomere and the rest of the DNA strand. However, the exact mechanism(s) by which all of these processes occur are far from being understood. It can be stated that stress and stress management are strongly connected to the biochemistry of the active substances bound up in the Sirtfoods. Additionally, chronic stress induces a situation where metabolism is well out of balance, or homeostatically challenged if you wish to be technical! Hence, if eating well can form part of an overall stress elimination (or at least management) program then consuming Sirtfoods may contribute to alleviating the genetic basis for ageing and could act as an insurance policy in terms of the health of the cell. Furthermore, cortisol_and other hormones are known to suppress the immune system and so stress, telomeres and Sirtfoods could collectively have a role in maintaining a defence against pathogens. The question is how we as individuals mediate between a normal and healthy stress response and a chronic, constant and consistent stress response. Intertwined with this question is the role of consuming a Sirt food rich diet in keeping stress levels down and the immune system functioning. Hence a further strand of Sirt food consumption is to reduce such symptoms but diet alone is not going to provide a person with space they need to deal with their stress. I mean let us be clear all the healthy eating in the world is not of itself going to fix the stresses caused by a consistently punishing work schedule or fix the relationship problems which are known to be caused by a work life balance that is skewed in the wrong direction, (i.e. toward work in case you were wondering).

Chapter 7: A Concise History of Sirtfood Research

"Man Is What He Eats" Titus Lucretius Carus (99 BC – 55 BC) was a Roman poet and philosopher

The year 2008 is a convenient start date for providing a context for research into the biochemistry of Sirtuin foods and Sirtuin Activators. In this year GlaxoSmithKline (GSK) for the tidy sum of $720 million brought out a US biotechnology firm called Sirtris Pharmaceuticals. The company was founded in 2004 by a Harvard biology graduate named Brian Sinclair. The interest of GSK was piqued because Sirtrus Pharmaceuticals were researching the role of compounds such as resveratrol and other polyphenol compounds in SIRT protein activation. It is the polyphenols which are recognised to contribute to the free radical clean up outlined below. In particular GSK were interested in the efficacy of a compound they named SRT-501, which contains resveratrol as its active ingredient. This of course begs an obvious question, *"what is resveratrol?"*

The precise chemical name for resveratrol is 3,5,4'-trihydroxystilbene which is manufactured by many autotrophs (plants) as a normal part of their metabolism. For instance the aggressively invasive Japanese knotweed synthesis this polyphenolic compound as a fungicide, which protects its roots from attack. In terms of our diet resveratrol is found in the skin of red grapes and so is helpfully found in copious amounts in all forms of red wine. Hurrah! It is also found in peanuts, dark chocolate and blue berries. Helpfully, all of these foods contain many of the vitamins (A through to K) and trace minerals (such as Iron and potassium), thus the healthy living benefits are self-evident and the potential efficacy of resveratrol an equally important bonus. In essence you can feel better about having peanut butter on toast, munching on your favourite peanuts during the football as well as grating dark chocolate on your blue berry and bananas in your morning muesli. While you're at it, you can feel free to wash it all down with a wholly desirable glass of Rioja, maybe not with breakfast though. This is wonderfully convenient because it is the skin of fruits such as red grapes and berries are considered to be the most concentrated source of resveratrol.

The compound SRT 501 was of interest to GlaxoSmithKline because it is believed to have a role in activating the SIRT1 protein. One area of interest was in the in the treatment of multiple myelomas. This type of cancer arises from the blood plasma, which is the alkaline liquid through which nutrients and waste products are exchanged in the blood stream. Myeloma affects the white blood cells manufactured in the bone marrow (where red blood cells are also continually manufactured). Hence myeloma can affect the overall composition and therefore effectiveness of the blood as a transport medium. Myeloma has a particular affinity for the white plasma cells involved in the production of anti-bodies, which are the proteins found in the cells of immune system. Antibodies function by recognising the antigens of pathogenic bacteria as well as virus particles and then the immune system is stimulated to destroy them. In the case of virus particles (such as those which cause the common cold) the body must manufacture sufficient quantities of the antibody carrying cells before the immune system is itself overwhelmed. Also known as immunoglobulins these antibodies are produced by white plasma cells on instruction from the T and B-cells of the immune system. Hence the plasma cells are crucial for a robust immune response and because these cells are manufactured in many bone marrow sites, myeloma can rapidly spread, hence the prefix "multiple". A person suffering from multiple myelomas has a severely degraded immune system. Thus, biological agents which would normally be harmless (or dealt with very quickly) can present a real danger to the health of the person. In effect the genetic make-up of the cells is changed such that they only manufacture a single anti-body called para-protein which has no known beneficial function. The presence of para protein is used to test for the presence of multiple myelomas. In many ways researching resveratrol is an example of a journey into the dark heart of the human condition.

Science is a human enterprise and despite it being one of the greatest achievements of our species scientists are not infallible and the literature is replete with instances of temptation and plain old scientific fraud fuelled by corruption. For example consider the U.S surgeon Dipak Das who in 2012 was found to have falsified data in 145 separate instances. Consequently said data was retracted including extensive work on the role of resveratrol in the treatment of heart disease. A further factor is the metabolism of resveratrol itself, the compound easily passes from the intestines to the liver. However, only about 1% of any ingested amount actually makes it to the blood stream. The compound is rapidly broken down and may well be converted to other substances before it can be transported to sites where it may express its potential benefits. Such poor bio-availability contrasts markedly with the action of resveratrol in vitro (outside the body) where it is applied to populations of micro-organisms in concentrations that have yet to be achieved in any clinical trial. At the time of writing the only way to obtain to obtain these kinds of dose levels is in the form of supplements.

The promotion of these supplements almost exclusively focuses on their purported cosmetic benefits. Such marketing has absolutely nothing to do with the transport and metabolism of resveratrol and everything to do with exploiting insecurity. Without a doubt these spurious claims ought to be categorically rejected. It is then unsurprising that research concerning the efficacy of synthetic derivatives of resveratrol continues apace. The question as to whether such derivatives should form part of a normal balanced diet will doubtless continue to present itself. As the reader can infer I am not a fan of certain supplements, however, it is not for me to preach, it is for the reader to make an informed choice. No matter your opinion, no supplement should be consumed without the knowledge or consent of your doctor. All of these indicators pertaining to the efficacy of resveratrol in human beings can be broken down into two basic suppositions. Either resveratrol is so potent that even tiny amounts garner physiological effects or that these effects are down to other metabolic factors that we have yet to determine. Concurrently, whether resveratrol and the other polyphenols have a role in chemo-prevention is a long way from being established.

In 2010 GlaxoSmithKline (GSK) ceased all clinical trials which used SRT-501 as an agent to counter the effects of multiple myelomas. In short it just didn't work and caused wholly undesirable side effects ranging from renal (kidney) failure to vomiting and diarrhoea, which then lead to dehydration. Clearly, just what you need when you are suffering from cancer. Subsequently, it has been shown that resveratrol is not shy when it comes to bonding to receptors and the active sites of many enzymes. Meaning it can have direct impacts on biochemical processes which may not benefit the person who has ingested too much of the chemical. In 2013 GSK shut down the subsidiary that it paid so much to acquire. This does not mean that research into Sirtuin Activators is dead and buried, quite the opposite, the potential is huge. As of 2015

GSK is continuing to research the efficacy of other plant based drugs. On top of all of this it must be remembered that we are talking about diet and not supplements. Many of the unpleasant side effects and other negative impacts which have occurred have been because the concentrations ingested have been so high. In other words the active ingredient has behaved as a toxin which the body will seek to remove by any means at its disposal. Research is now focusing on the metabolic pathways in which the chemicals in side Sirtfoods are thought to function. A key focus of the science is to find molecules which are much more selective than resveratrol and do not provoke side effects. In terms of chemo-prevention no such molecule that specifically targets the Sirtuin Activators (SA's) has been discovered. Red wine contains anything up to 14mg of resveratrol per litre and you must feel free to enjoy a glass of your favourite brew of alcoholic grape juice. Just don't expect it to be a panacea cure for undesirable biological conditions.

So what is the future of research into Sirt proteins and their activating chemicals? Well put simply it's bright and like all good science it's self-regulating and it learns from its mistakes. In this frame Sirtfood research ought to be viewed as an example of science operating at its best. The reader must appreciate that much of the literature published and science being conducted is occurring at the limits of our knowledge in this area. The next big discovery in the field could quite literally be around the next corner. The SIRT proteins are known to be most active when the body is metabolising within its optimal limits (homeostasis). This fact should imply that cellular health will be maintained and diseases such as cancer, diabetes and all the other conditions associated with western diet are nullified. Much of the current research and likely future research on Sirt proteins and their activators is concerned with using diet as a preventative measure to assuage these negative biological conditions. For instance a compound is known as SIRT2104, (which seems to activate SIRT1) is undergoing what are termed *"initial safety studies"*. This is scientific parlance for the safety trials that are carried on volunteers who in this case are prone to type 2 diabetes and inflammatory diseases. The same compound has been postulated to have a role in treating aspects of crohn's disease and its equally unpleasant bed fellow IBS (Irritable Bowl Syndrome). However, please don't hold your breath; there is still a long way to go. Which gives us a helpful moment to reiterate that where ever possible prevention is better than cure?

Fundamentally there are 7 inter-related strands of research pertaining to the biochemistry andactivation of the SIRT proteins. One recent development concerns research published in 2014 which focuses on the SIRT6. It is known that the SIRT6 enzyme inhibits tumor growth in the liver and colon of laboratory animals. However, the same protein has been observed to promote the growth of skin cancer cells because it has been shown to activate the enzymes which induce skin tumor growth. In other words there is a possibility that exposure to UV-B radiation could negate the action of SIRT6, at least as far as the skin is concerned. The SIRT 6 enzyme does have an implicit role in protecting DNA from genomic instability but this research appears to indicate that this efficacy varies between tissue types and can be disrupted by external factors. The point here is that if you are going to catch some rays, you had better do it with moderation and especially be careful not to burn. The same research demonstrated that when laboratory mice were genetically engineered to not express SIRT6 the incidence of skin cancer was significantly reduced. The mode of action in this context concerns the relationship between SIRT6 and an enzyme known as COX-2. This enzyme is responsible for skin inflammation, cellular reproduction (mitosis) and it is known to extend the life span of skin cells. These processes are inextricably bound up in the proliferation of cancer cells. In this particular set of experiments when SIRT6 levels were increased so did skin cancer, when SIRT 6 levels were reduced so did the incidence of the cancer cells. In other words there is a direct correlation between the two variables. The research supposes that exposure to UV-B light promotes the activity of SIRT6 in skin cells and that this activity increase the production of the COX-2 enzyme. Overall, this single piece of research underpins the complexity of the science involved in SIRT protein science. On the one hand we know more about the onset of skin cancer, on the other science needs to establish ways to inhibit this expression without disrupting its other functions in the body.

Chapter 8: A Final Word

"Let thy food be thy medicine and thy medicine be thy food" Hippocrates (460-377B.C.)

Some form of regular exercise is essential to achieving any degree of weight loss; now this does not have to mean joining a gym or pumping iron every day. It means riding your push bike or walking to work and leaving the car at home whenever you can. Clearly, you should consult your doctor or health practitioner for advice but I can guarantee that he or she will ask you about your eating habits. Your job is to take heed and follow as best you can their instructions. The trick is to maintain a healthy balance between eating, metabolism and exercise. Irrespective of an individual context the fact remains, if excess fat is allowed to accumulate then the person is sure to become *"overweight"* if things slip further the person may become a contributor to the *"global obesity epidemic"* alluded to elsewhere in this text. The more you exercise or the more active you are, the more carbohydrates and fats are "burned off" in the mitochondria. The reader should not be left with the impression that one particular aspect of their diet will definitely prevent the onset of cancer or indeed any other negative biological occurrence. In other words do not rush out and buy bags of green tea and expect not to develop cancer if you are not implementing other positive changes to your life style. Having stated that, the potential benefits of eating Sirtfoods as part of your normal healthy eating routine in this book cannot be understated. The substances thought to activate the SIRT proteins are, at their simplest, chemicals derived from the food that we eat. We obtain these chemicals through digestion and they are then used in their entirety to drive our metabolism. In other words all those lovely colours that you see in all the food you have ever eaten no matter the forms in which you ingest are made of chemicals. The chemicals which keep us alive are atoms of carbon, hydrogen, nitrogen, oxygen, phosphorous and sulphur which are arranged and chemically bonded together to form the compounds we eat. We also consume vitamins and minerals which are by and large made of the same atoms as well as fibre and water. In other words every substance that we eat and then digest has some sort of metabolic function. Of course it's self-evident that they will influence the biochemistry of the SIRT proteins and will be enhanced if they are regularly stocked up with the molecules we need to ingest irrespective of our knowledge of their existence. To me, that says Job done!

This book is the culmination of a long and sometimes painful journey from health to fitness. I had to completely re-evaluate what I thought I knew about food and even our society and the way it functions (that's for another book). It can be very challenging to face off old beliefs that are engrained from an early age about food. During this journey one of the most startling discoveries I made was that your regular MD has very little knowledge about diet and health. They seem to know the basics like everyone does but they never have time to specialise. It's much easier to treat a symptom with pharmaceuticals than to really understand and prevent the cause of the illness. I'm not looking for a bandage or a pill from my doctor; I want knowledge that prevents illness in the first place. Good health and ill health can be promoted by your own body; it just needs the correct fuel in the form of nutrition. If you eat dead food that's overly processed and full of additives and chemicals you will slowly starve your cells of nutrition and then the worst nightmares can and often will happen. The old hippy adage comes to mind "treat your body like a temple" or in today's zeitgeist "treat your body like a sports car". Make sure you have only the best quality fuel/food working in your body, your body deserves it. During our brief time here our bodies have a lot of work to do so treat it well. J. Hodges

12 Easy SIRT FOOD Recipes To Get You Started

FROM VIDDA KITCHEN

The twelve recipes contained here will hopefully inspire some ideas of your own on how to incorporate Sirt Foods into your diet. Some of these meal ideas have become a mainstay and favorite within our own personal nutritional regime. It's hard to think of breakfast without the 'Spicy Toast' and a Superhero Smoothie at least three times a week.

A firm favorite among our friends is the Vegan Chocolate Mousse. I always have to show the recipe and ingredients to prove that the mousse is not made with dairy products, it's that good.

The secret is, don't over complicate or over think your diet. Keep adding good quality and nutrient rich foods. Of course, it's very important to identify and discard the hidden toxins and dangers in your current 'mainstream' diet. This will take research and painful realisations to get the most health benefits from a dietary change on the path to a healthier you. I hope the research you've just read in this book has helped you decide that a highly nutritous diet full of Sirt foods is the best preventative medicine you can give yourself.

It's not always easy but the rewards are undeniable. Before you know it, as you regain your vitality and taste for 'real' food you'll notice that your taste buds and olfactory functions will have changed. The foods that were part of your unhealthy diet will all of a sudden not register with you as something you'd want in your body. It's almost as if the body wakes up and starts protecting you from the dangers out there. The cleaner your diet becomes the better it works.

Your body is going to thank you a million times over in both subtle and profound ways, enjoy the journey, be adventurous, constantly question your food intake and stay healthy.

Superhero Green Smoothie

Not for the faint hearted!

Serves 4 (Makes 2 litres)

Ingredients:

1 tbsp wheatgrass powder (optional)

1 tbsp spirulina (optional)

1 tbsp Bee Pollen (optional)

1 tbsp freshly ground flaxseed (optional)

1 tsp cinnamon

1 sheet of Nori Roll (seaweed)

1 stick of rhubarb (cut in chunks)

1 medium ripe pear (cut in quarters)

1 un-waxed lemon with skin (cut in quarters)

1 washed kiwi with skin (cut in half)

1 ripe banana (chopped)

3 - 4 cm piece of ginger with skin (cut in small chunks)

3 dandelion flowers

10 dandelion leaves

10 stems of goose grass

5 small heads of purple sprouting / broccoli

3 Cavolo Nero (kale) leaves

3 small cabbage leaves

1.5 pints of cold filtered water (or coconut water)

Method:

Throw all the ingredients in your smoothie maker ensuring that the supplement powders and pollen are in the middle. Top up with water, place the lid on and whizz away until well blended and you achieve a smooth consistency. If it is too thick for your taste, you can always add more coconut or filtered water.

The Choco-Mint Smoothie

For a simpler smoothie recipe try these ingredients.

Serves 4 (Makes 2 litres)

Ingredients:

1/2 bag of Baby Spinach

Large Handful of fresh Mint

1 Pear

1 Green Apple

1 Lemon with skin

1 ripe Banana

1 chunk of Ginger (size optional)

3 tbsp Cacao Nibs

1tsp Cinnamon

1 tbsp Wheatgrass powder

1 tbsp Spirulina

1 tbsp Bee Pollen

2 tbsp Chia Seeds

Large tbsp Cold Pressed Coconut Oil

Top up with filtered water & blend

Method:

Chop and put all the ingredients in your smoothie maker, top with water, place lid on and whiz away until well blended and you achieve a smooth consistency. Add more water if too thick for your taste.

The Taste of India - Spicy Toast

This is a really simple breakfast or snack that's full of antioxidants and natural fat burning chemicals and the Turmeric is a powerful Sirtfood.

Serves 1

Ingredients:

2 slices of Crusty Rye Bread or dark rye bread, toasted

Extra Virgin Olive Oil or Hemp Oil

Turmeric

Black Pepper

Himalayan Pink Salt (Or Sea Salt)

Cayenne Pepper

Sliced onions

Cherry or Vine Tomatoes Mung Bean Sprouts

Method:

Drizzle Extra Virgin Olive Oil on your toast. Alternatively, I like to use Hemp Oil which is very high in protein. Sprinkle Turmeric, Cayenne Pepper, Black Pepper & Salt to taste. Slice some sweet cherry tomatoes (or a Vine tomato) and add some sprouts (Mung Beans or Lentils).

Of course, if you want it simple, just toast your bread, add the oil and the spices. I warn you, this can be addictive. I call it Rainbow Toast.

VIDDA Granola

Delicious as a snack on its own or served in a bowl with yogurt or milk (almond or hemp)

Serves 6 – 8

Ingredients:

200 grams of rolled oat & barley

125 grams mixed nuts (almonds, walnuts, hazelnuts)

100 grams of mixed seeds (flaxseeds, sesame, pumpkin, sunflower, poppy)

50 grams of desiccated coconut

1 teaspoons of ground cinnamon

125 grams of dried fruit (flame raisins, golden raisins & cranberries)

3 tablespoons of organic honey

2 tablespoon of extra virgin olive oil.

Method:

Preheat oven to 180°C (350°F / Gas mark 4)

Mix and place all your dry ingredients (except for the dried fruits) on a baking try. Drizzle with olive oil and honey and

stir. Place in the oven for approximately 30 minutes, stirring approximately every 7 minutes. When the granola turns to a golden colour, remove from the oven. Stir in the dried fruit and leave it to cool down. Once completely cold, store it in an airtight container.

Sirt Food Tip: Granola Layer Crunch

Find a nice serving glass (a tumbler will be great) and start with a layer of fresh berries, followed by a layer of granola and a layer of natural yogurt (repeat as many times as you want / need to fill your serving dish). Top all off with a generous sprinkle of cinnamon and a drizzle of honey.

Butternut Squash and Ginger Soup

Serves 4

Ingredients:

2 tbsp Extra Virgin Olive Oil

1 large onion, finely chopped

3 garlic cloves (crushed)

2 - 3 cm piece of fresh ginger (grated)

1 sweet red pepper 1 kg Butternut squash (peeled, deseeded and chopped into chunks)

700 ml Vegetable stock

Handful of pumpkin seeds

Method:

Heat the olive oil in a large saucepan, then gently cook the onions and pepper for 5 minutes or until onions are soft but not coloured. Add the garlic and ginger and cook for 1 minute before adding the pumpkin. Carry on cooking for 8-10 minutes, stirring occasionally until it starts to soften and turn golden.

Pour the stock into the pan, then season with salt and pepper. Bring to the boil, then simmer for approximately 10 minutes until the squash is very soft. Remove the saucepan from cooker and let it cool down a bit before pureeing with a hand blender. For a super velvety consistency, you can push the soup through a fine sieve into another pan. While the soup is cooking, dry toast in a pan a handful of pumpkin seeds (careful not to burn them). Serve soup scattered with the pumpkin seeds (fresh parsley or cress) and a slice of crusty spelt loaf.

Sirt Food Tip: Sprinkle the soup with cayenne pepper, turmeric or a little bit of curry powder.

Sweet and Spicy Rice

This is a great dish on its own or served as a side dish. A great way to use leftover rice. Quick and easy to make

Serves 3 - 4

Ingredients:

225 gr. brown rice (500 gr., if cooked)

100 gr. sultanas

1 large onion

85 gr. pumpkin seeds

2 tsp cinnamon powder

1 tsp curry powder

1/2 tsp Himalayan pink salt

1.5 tbsp extra Virgin Olive oil

Method:

Cook the rice following cooking instructions on the packet. Drain and put aside

Dry toast the pumpkin seeds lightly in a large frying pan. Set aside.

Soak the sultanas in a bowl with lukewarm water for approximately 2 minutes. Drain well and set aside.

Whilst the rice is cooking, finely cut the onion

Heat the oil in the same frying pan and cook the onions for about 5 minutes until they are soft and golden. Add the cooked rice and stir for a couple of minutes on a medium-low heat.

Add the drained sultanas, toasted pumpkin seeds, curry, cinnamon and salt to the mix and combine well.

Check and adjust seasoning. Serve straight away.

Crunchy Living Sprout Sandwich

Serves 1

Ingredients:

1 Flaxseed rye roll

Extra virgin olive oil

Cayenne pepper

Himalayan Pink salt (or Sea Salt)

Chopped onion

Cucumber

1 vine tomato (sliced)

Mung bean & sunflower sprouts

Method:

Slice roll and drizzle oil on both sides. Then add spices followed by chopped onion,

cucumber, tomato, and sprouts.

Wild Garlic and Chilli Oil Green Salad

Serves 1

Ingredients:

Lambs lettuce

Rocket leaves

1 stick of celery, chopped

1 small red pepper, sliced

1 small onion, chopped

6 halved cherry tomatoes

1/3 medium cucumber, sliced

5 wild garlic leaves with flowers, roughly chopped

Small handful of Mung beans sprouts

Extra Virgin Olive Oil

Apple Cider Vinegar

Turmeric

Cayenne Pepper

Black Pepper

Himalayan pink salt

Method:

Mix all ingredients together in a bowl. Drizzle with chili oil, apple cider vinegar, turmeric, cayenne pepper, black pepper, and salt.

Stewed Apple and Rhubarb Coolie

Absolutely delicious with a dollop of natural yoghurt or as a crumble filling. You can also serve it with granola or muesli.

Serves 6

Ingredients:

6 sticks of rhubarb

2 Bramley apples

3 cm piece of freshly grated ginger (more if you enjoy the

taste)

3 cloves

2 cinnamon sticks

Honey, to taste

1/2 cup of filtered water

Method:

Peel and chop the apples. If rhubarb stalks are too fibrous, peel the strings off. Then chop up. Place the fruit in a saucepan with the water. Peel and grate the ginger and add it to the fruit, along with the cloves and the cinnamon sticks. Stir frequently to avoid sticking. Once the fruit starts to soften up add the honey. When the fruit is soft, remove the lid from the pan and let the liquid reduce. Serve hot or cold.

Surprise Vegan Chocolate Mousse

The surprise being that this delicious and velvety chocolate dessert is extremely good for you and made with avocado!

Serves 3

Ingredients:

1 tbsp of coconut oil

1 ripe avocado

Rind of 1 medium orange (finely grated)

Juice from 1 medium orange (add a bit at a time

until desired consistency is achieved)

2 large tablespoons of raw cacao powder

2 tbsp of organic honey (add more if you have a

sweet tooth)

Method:

Melt the coconut oil in a heatproof bowl set over a pan of hot water. Add the avocado flesh, the orange juice and rind and whizz with a hand blender until smooth. Add the cacao powder and the honey and whizz again until very smooth. You can always add more cocoa powder honey or orange for stronger flavours.

Put the mousse into individual dishes and chill in the fridge for a minimum of 1 hour. Serve with a selection of berries of your liking (raspberries, blackberries, strawberries or blueberries).

Alternatively, go the extra mile and present it in a large wine glass over a base of Date and Coconut Crust (see recipe below):

Date and Coconut Crust

1 cup of shredded coconut

1 cup of walnuts 1/4 teaspoon of Himalayan pink salt

1/4 cup pitted dates

Place the coconut, walnuts, and salt in a food processor and process until coarsely ground. Add the dates and process until it starts to stick together and looks like coarse crumbs

Sirt-Slow

Serves 2 as a side dish or 1 as a main

Ingredients:

2 carrots

¼ white cabbage (sliced)

1 small onion

1 apple

1 handful of sultanas or raisins

1 handful of pumpkin seeds

1 handful of cress or mixed sprouts, such as broccoli, mung bean, sunflower

Small handful of fresh mint

Method:

Dry toast the pumpkin seeds lightly in a large frying pan. Set aside.

Soak the sultanas in a bowl with lukewarm water for approximately 2 minutes. Drain well and set aside.

Peel and grate the carrots.

Finely slice the onion, cabbage

Finely chop the fresh mint

Core and dice the apple

Mix all ingredients in a large bowl. Season with pink Himalayan salt, black pepper, and a drizzle of olive oil. Alternatively, you can make the following <u>healthy nutty dressing</u>:

- 200g of raw cashew nuts

- 1 tsp of mustard

- Juice of half a large lemon (add more to taste)

- 150 ml of filtered water

- Place all ingredients in a blender until you achieve a smooth creamy consistency. If required, add more water or lemon juice

Veggie Sprout Sweet Potato Soup

Serves 4

Ingredients:

2 tbsp Extra Virgin Olive Oil

1 large onion, finely chopped

2 garlic cloves (crushed)

5-6 Brussel Sprouts

1 large sweet potato (cut into cubes)

150gr asparagus (chopped)

100 gr closed cup mushrooms (sliced)

700 ml Vegetable stock

Handful of mung bean sprouts (or other, such as broccoli, alfalfa)

Method:

Heat the olive oil in a large saucepan over a medium heat, then gently add the onions and fry for approximately 5 minutes or until soft.

Add the garlic and cook for 1 minute before adding the sweet potato, brussel sprouts mushrooms and asparagus. Carry on cooking for 3 -5 minutes, stirring occasionally.

Pour the stock into the pan, then season to taste with salt and pepper, as needed. Bring to the boil, then simmer for approximately 10 minutes until the vegetables are cooked.

Serve with a handful of mung bean sprouts and a sprinkle of turmeric and/or cayenne pepper.

Our Top Dozen Favourite Sirt Foods from VIDDA Kitchen

The Health Benefits of Turmeric

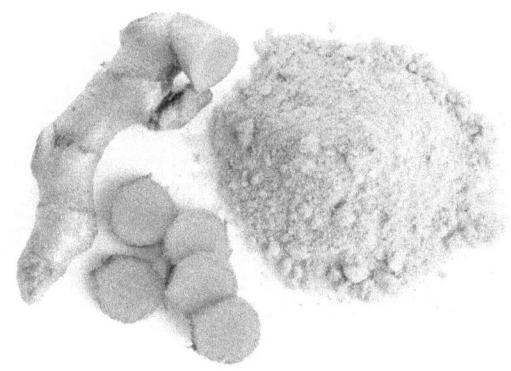

Often called the World's greatest Superfood.

Compounds are called Curcuminoids, the most important of which is Curcumin has powerful anti-inflammatory properties and very strong antioxidants.

Inflammation is now scientifically linked to nearly all chronic disease.

When taken with Black Pepper which contains the compound Peperine the absorption level of the powerful Curcumin rises by up to 2000%.

Curcumin increases levels of the brain hormone BDNF.

BDNF increases the growth of new neurones fighting various degenerative processes in the brain

Curcumin improves the function of the endothelium and is a potent anti-inflammatory agent and antioxidant protecting against several factors conducive to heart disease.

Current research is showing that Curcumin has a powerful effect in destroying and halting the spread of all types of cancer cells.

Curcumin can cross the blood-brain barrier and has been shown to lead to various improvements in the pathological process of Alzheimer's disease by clearing the build-up of protein tangles called Amyloid plaques in the brain.

Studies show that curcumin can help treat symptoms of arthritis and is in some cases more effective than anti-inflammatory drugs.

Curcumin is as effective as Prozac in alleviating the symptoms of depression.

Nutrients & Phytonutrients:

Dietary Fibre, Protein

Fatty Acids - Omega 3, Omega 6

Vitamins - Vitamin C, Vitamin E (Alpha Tocopherol), Vitamin K, Niacin, Vitamin B6, Folate, Choline, Betaine

Minerals - Calcium, Iron, Magnesium, Phosphorus, Potassium, Sodium, Zinc, Manganese, Selenium

Sterols – Phytosterols

The Health Benefits of Walnuts

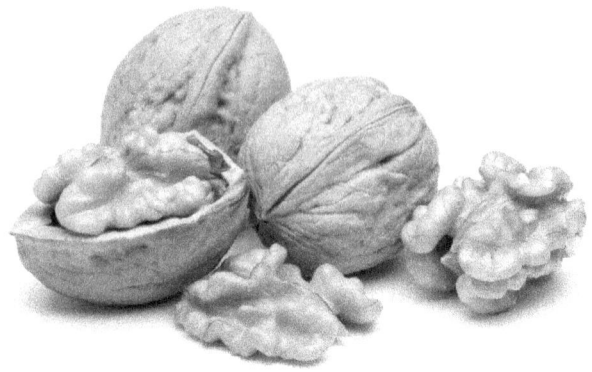

Rich source of polyunsaturated fats, especially the omega-6 fatty acid called linoleic acid which has been identified as a powerful anti-inflammatory and especially beneficial for heart health. It also helps regulate the composition of blood fats.

Walnuts are one of the richest dietary sources of antioxidants. These include ellagic acid, ellagitannins, catechin, and melatonin.

Walnuts have several bioactive compounds such as Phytosterols, Gamma-tocopherol, Omega-3fatty acids, Ellagic acid, antioxidant polyphenols and research is starting to show that with regular consumption these have potential cancer-fighting properties, especially with breasts, prostate, colon and kidneys cancers.

Many studies are showing that Walnuts may improve brain function and slow the progression of Alzheimer's disease.

While Walnuts are considered a superfood, some people should avoid them because of the dangers of nut allergy. They may also reduce mineral absorption in some of the population.

Nutrients & Phytonutrients:

Dietary Fibre, Protein

Fatty Acids - High levels of Omega 3, Omega 6

Vitamins - Vitamin A, Vitamin C, Vitamin E (Alpha Tocopherol), Vitamin K, Niacin, Vitamin B6, Riboflavin, Thiamin, Folate, Pantothenic Acid, Choline, Betaine

Minerals - Calcium, Iron, Magnesium, Phosphorus, Potassium, Sodium, Zinc, Copper, Manganese, Selenium

Sterols – Phytosterols

The Health Benefits of Celery

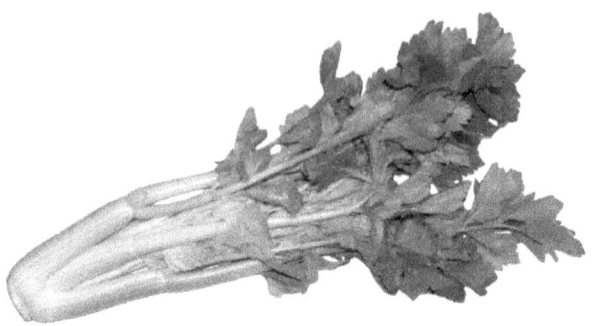

Celery reduces inflammation aiding in reduction of joint pains, lung infections, asthma, and even acne.

The mineral magnesium helps reduce stress and also aids sleep if eaten before bedtime

Celery regulates the body's alkaline balance.

Celery has a high water and soluble fibre content thus aiding in regular bowel movement

Celery contains natural organic salt (sodium) which is essential for a healthy nervous system.

One large stalk of celery can deliver up to 10 percent of your daily need for Vitamin A, a group of nutrients that protects the eyes and prevents age-related degeneration of vision.

The active compound called phthalides in celery has been proven to boost circulatory health and reduce high blood pressure.

Two pheromones in celery—androstenone and androstenol—boost your arousal levels and can improve sexual performance.

Research conducted at the University of Illinois show that a powerful flavonoid in celery, called luteolin, inhibits the growth of cancer cells, especially in the pancreas and also may inhibit the growth of breast cancer.

Nutrients & Phytonutrients:

Dietary Fibre, Protein

Fatty Acids - High levels of Omega 6

Vitamins - Vitamin A, Vitamin C, Vitamin E (Alpha Tocopherol), Vitamin K, Riboflavin, Niacin, Vitamin B6, Folate, Pantothenic Acid, Choline, Betaine

Minerals - Calcium, Iron, Magnesium, Phosphorus, Potassium, Sodium, Zinc, Manganese, Selenium, Fluoride.

Sterols – Phytosterols

The Health Benefits of Strawberries

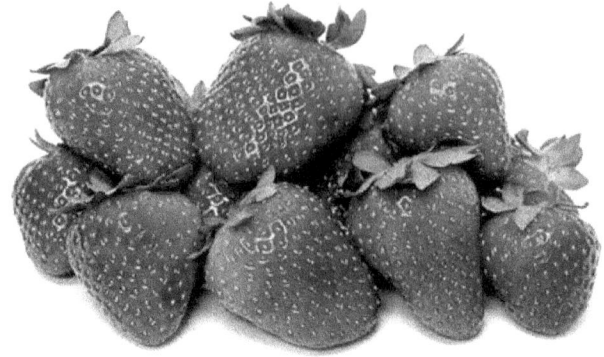

The chemical that gives the famous red colouring contains anthocyanins which help burn stored fat.

If eaten daily anthocyanins have been shown to improve short-term memory by 100% in eight weeks.

Extremely low in calories and high in fibre.

Strawberries are an effective and powerful anti-inflammatory by lowering blood levels of C-reactive protein (CRP).

The Flavonoids which are responsible for the colour and flavour of strawberries help lower the risk for cardiovascular disease.

Strawberries promote bone health because of they contain levels of potassium, vitamin K and magnesium.

Studies show freeze-dried strawberry powder may help prevent human oesophageal cancer.

Regular consumption of Strawberries may lower the risk of macular degeneration, a condition resulting in vision loss.

Strawberries are loaded with Biotin which promotes strong hair and nails. Also, they contain the antioxidant ellagic acid which helps protect the elastic fibres in the epidermis and prevent saggy skin.

CAUTION: people with kidney or gallbladder condition should avoid strawberries because of the oxalates that may interfere with the absorption of calcium.

Nutrients & Phytonutrients:

Dietary Fibre, Protein

Fatty Acids - Omega 3, Omega 6.

Vitamins - Vitamin A, Vitamin C, Vitamin E (Alpha Tocopherol), Vitamin K, Niacin, Vitamin B6, Folate, Pantothenic Acid, Choline, Betaine

Minerals – Calcium, Iron, Magnesium, Phosphorus, Potassium, Sodium, Zinc, Copper, Manganese, Selenium, Fluoride

Sterols – Phytosterols

The Health Benefits of Watercress

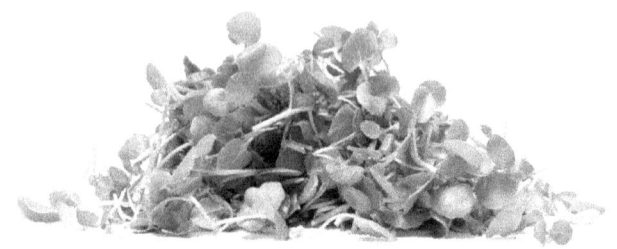

Rich in vitamin C aiding cell regeneration, liver health, and immune system helping fight infection and viruses.

Contains Phenethyl Isothiocyanate which helps detoxify the liver and is a known carcinogen.

Rich in Iodine - essential for thyroid function.

B6 helps prevent memory loss.

Watercress helps the release of bile from the gall bladder which aids the digestion of fat.

Helps break up kidney & bladder stones.

Keeps heart and skin healthy.

Nutrients & Phytonutrients:

Vitamin B3, Vitamin B6, Vitamin C, Carotennoids, Calcium, Iron, Magnesium, Fibre

The Health Benefits of Green tea

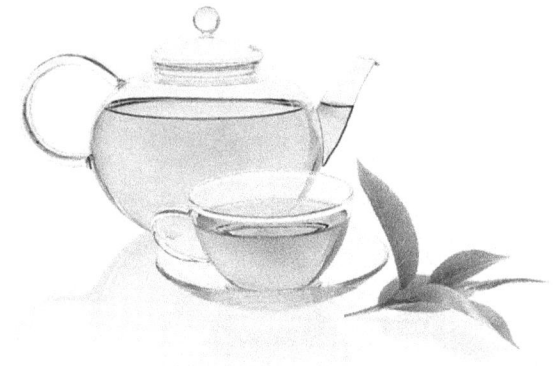

Inhibits Cancer cell growth.

Improves the ratio between good and bad Cholesterol.

Protects against Heart Disease & Heart Attaches.

Increasing Metabolism & increases Fat Oxidation.

Helps prevent Diabetes.

Antiviral properties.

Increases Brain Activity

Regulates Blood Pressure.

Treats Rheumatoid Arthritis.

Rich in Tannins that helps skin stress.

High in Polyphenols aiding protection from UVA & UVB sun rays.

A specific type of Polyphenol called Catechins helps kill acne-causing skin bacteria.

The Health Benefits of Nutritional Yeast

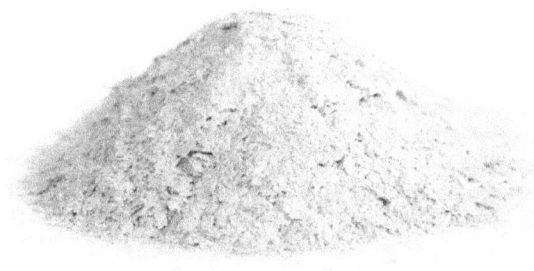

Nutritional Yeast is one of the few non-animal sources of B-12.

Rich in folic acid plus multiple other nutrients and amino acids.

Rich in B vitamins, including B12.

It is a great source of 18 amino acids, protein, folic acid, biotin and other vitamins.

It is also rich in 15 minerals including iron, magnesium, phosphorus, zinc, chromium, & selenium.

It is grown on beet sugar and molasses, fermented & dried so it is gluten free.

It has a nutty, cheesy taste and makes a great addition to soups, pasta, salads, sandwiches, and my favourite, sprinkled on Rye Bread with a little Virgin Olive Oil and Cayenne Pepper

The Health Benefits of Kale

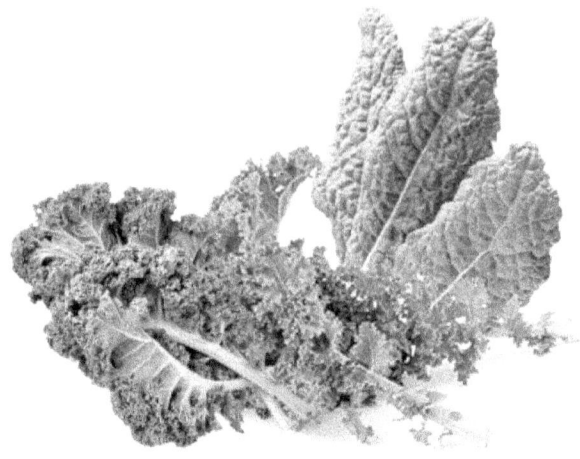

Kale is amongst the most nutrient-dense foods on the planet.

High in Antioxidants such as Quercetin and Kaempferol.

Anti-viral & Anti-Bacterial.

Reduces Cholesterol.

Overall Skin health.

Daily consumption fights and prevents most Cancers.

Strengthens Heart muscle.

Anti-depressant.

Good dietary source of Vitamin C and Vitamin B6.

One of the highest sources of Vitamin K.

Protects eyesight.

High in Sulforaphane.

Low Glycemic Index.

Antioxidants that may help Prevent Alzheimer's Disease and Dementia.

Boost immune system.

Super Tip: If cooking for preparation, steaming or boiling pre-chop and leave for 40 minutes to activate and keep the cancer-fighting Sulforaphane. Or alternatively, add 1/2 tsp of mustard powder (myrosinase enzymes) sprinkled onto the kale as a condiment. Horse Radish or Wasabi will also do the same job.

Nutrients & Phytonutrients:

Dietary Fibre, Protein

Fatty Acids - Omega 3, Omega 6

Vitamins - Niacin, Pantothenic acid, Riboflavin, Thiamin, Vitamin A, Vitamin C, Vitamin K, Vitamin B6, Folate, Minerals, Calcium, Iron, Magnesium, Phosphorus, Potassium, Sodium, Zinc, Copper, Manganese, Selenium

The Health Benefits of Blueberries

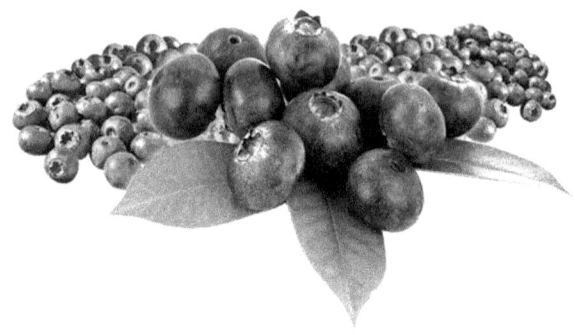

Phytonutrients function both as antioxidants and as anti-inflammatory compounds in the body.

Protection from Cardiovascular Disease.

Improved Cognitive function including memory.

Blood sugar regulation, useful for treating Type 2 Diabetes.

Anthocyanins found in Blueberries help protect the retina in the eye from sunlight and oxidative stress. Studies show increased protection from breast cancer, colon cancer, oesophagal cancer, and cancers of the small intestine.

Nutrients & Phytonutrients:

Phytonutrients: Anthocyanins, Malvidins, Delphinidins, Pelargonidins, Cyanidins, Peonidins

Hydroxycinnamic acid: Caffeic acids, Ferulic acids, Coumaric acids, Hydroxybenzoic acids, Gallic acids

Protocatechuic acids: Flavonols, Kaempferol, Quercetin, Myricetin

Other phenol-related phytonutrients: Pterostilbene, Resveratrol

The Health Benefits of Olives

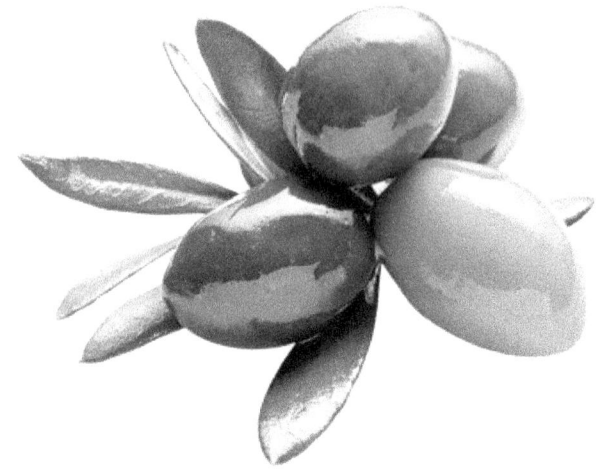

Olives eliminate excess cholesterol in the blood.

Olives control blood pressure.

Olives are a source of dietary fibre as an alternative to fruits and vegetables.

Olives are a great source of Vitamin E.

Olives act as an antioxidant, protecting cells.

Olives reduce the effects of degenerative diseases like Alzheimer's, benign and malignant tumours, including less serious varicose veins and cavities.

Olives help prevent blood clots that could lead to a myocardial infarction or deep vein thrombosis (DVT).

Olives protect cell membranes against diseases like cancer.

Olives are a great protection against anaemia.

Olives enhance fertility and reproductive system.

Olives play an important role in maintaining a healthy immune system, especially during oxidative stress and chronic viral diseases and much, much more.

Nutrients & Phytonutrients:

Phytonutrients: Carotene-B, Crypto-xanthin-B, Lutein-zeaxanthin, Phytosterols

Vitamins: Niacin, Pantothenic acid, Pyridoxine, Riboflavin, Thiamin, Vitamin A, Vitamin C, Vitamin E, Vitamin K

Minerals: Calcium, Copper, Iron, Magnesium, Manganese, Phosphorus, Selenium, Zinc

Electrolytes: Sodium, Potassium.

The Health Benefits of Garlic

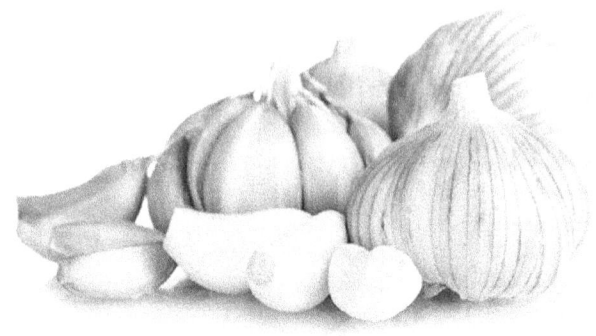

Great dietary way to increase Selenium.

Proven to reduce Blood Pressure.

Anti-viral.

Anti-Bacterial.

Reduces Cholesterol.

Aids Digestion (take on empty stomach 30 mins before eating).

Overall Skin health.

Daily consumption fights and prevents most Cancers.

Strengthens Heart muscle.

Controls Blood sugar.

Treats Skin problems, such as rashes and spots when applied topically.

Good dietary source of Vitamin C and Vitamin B6.

Rich source of Manganese.

Low Glycemic Index.

Antioxidants that may help Prevent Alzheimer's Disease and Dementia.

Improves Athletic Performance.

Detoxify Heavy Metals from the Body.

Fight and prevents the Common Cold

Super Tip: Chop and slice and leave for 30 minutes before consumption to activate the SUPER sulphur compound called Allicin. Take with 1 teaspoon of Organic Honey if the taste is a problem.

Nutrients & Phytonutrients:

Dietary Fibre, Protein

Fatty Acids - Omega 3, Omega 6

Vitamins - Niacin, Pantothenic acid, Pyridoxine, Riboflavin, Thiamin, Vitamin A, Vitamin C, Vitamin E, Vitamin K, Vitamin B6, Folate, Choline

Minerals - Calcium, Iron, Magnesium, Phosphorus, Potassium, Sodium, Zinc, Copper, Manganese, Selenium

The Health Benefits of Blackberries

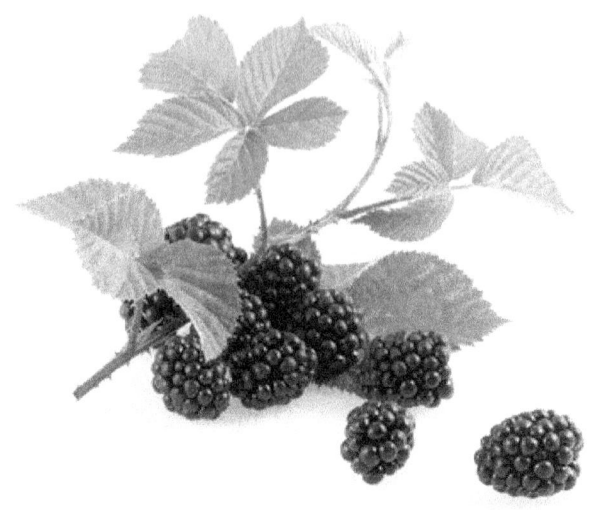

High amounts of phenolic flavonoid phytochemicals such as anthocyanins, ellagic acid, tannin, quercetin, gallic acid, cyanidins, pelargonidins, catechins, kaempferol, and salicylic acid Blackberries contain gallic acid, rutin and ellagic acid, compounds that may have antiviral and antibacterial properties

Improves oral health because of antiviral & antibacterial qualities.

Reduces Cholesterol.

Improves Skin health

Anti- Carcinogen.

Protects your cardiovascular system from disease

Good dietary source of Vitamin C and Vitamin B6.

Improve eye health.

Very low Glycemic Index.

Positive impact on motor and cognitive skills.

Boost immune system.

Nutrients & Phytonutrients:

High Dietary Fibre, Protein

Fatty Acids - Omega 3, Omega 6,

Vitamins - Niacin, Pantothenic acid, Riboflavin, Thiamin, Vitamin A, Vitamin C, Vitamin E (Alpha Tocopherol), Vitamin K, Vitamin B6, Folate

Minerals - Calcium, Iron, Magnesium, Phosphorus, Potassium, Sodium, Zinc, Copper, Manganese, Selenium

Before you go

Thank you for purchasing my book!

If you found this book interesting and enjoyed reading it, I would really appreciate a short **review on Amazon**. All of your feedback is valuable to me, as your comments and input will be taken on board to help me make this and future books even better.

I would love hearing what you have to say. Please leave me a helpful REVIEW on Amazon.

FREE Bonus Chapter: Volume 2 "The Medicine On Your Plate"

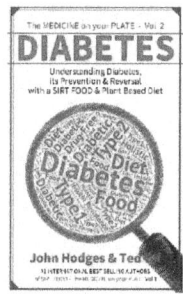

DIABETES: PREVENTION & REVERSAL with a SIRTFOOD & PLANT-BASED DIET (by John Hodges & Ted Gif)

Introduction: Diet & Diabetes

The first point to specify with this writing is that several charities and organisations will be mentioned throughout this Book. The reader needs to realise that neither yours truly or VIDDA Publishing have received any endorsements, sweeteners, brown paper bags or similar receptacles from these organisations I have presented their findings because the ethos (authority) exists to do so. Right, that's that dealt with!

This Book is designed to give the reader an overview of what diabetes actually is and how it can be treated. The text is not designed to second guess the medical professionals in the field but to present their core assertions in an objective, easy to digest and informative way. It is designed to empower and inspire those who have been diagnosed with Type 2 diabetes, by making absolutely clear that the condition can be reversed if the dietary and another advice contained herein is followed. I have no real authority to discuss the treatment for Type-one diabetes. The reason is simple I do not have the diagnosis, there is no history of it in my family and so I have sought to present in the writing the essential differences between the two conditions. I have also sought to present some of the latest scientific research in the field of Type one diabetes treatment. With this in mind, the reader is encouraged to follow the advice outlined in the last paragraph of this introduction. Toward the end of the SIRTFOODS book mention was made of the biochemistry of "diabetes" we shall be revisiting these terms and explaining the difference between type one and type two diabetes. The difference between the two conditions will be explained in chapter one, but at the outset, the reader may find it useful to see the two "types" as different conditions, at least in terms of their cause.

This book will not be considering gestational diabetes which as the term implies affects women who are pregnant but cannot produce enough insulin during the gestation period. This book will first and foremost present a case for preventing the onset of type two diabetes by paying attention to diet and exercise. It is this aspect that is highlighted in chapter two and the reader should be left under no illusions concerning the global scale of the diabetes epidemic. The third chapter will outline the individual and holistic nature of both prevention and cure for both forms of diabetes. The final chapter will present some of the more bizarre myths I came across whilst carrying out the research for this book. Furthermore, the last chapter will reiterate and recapitulate the key points made throughout the text but apply them to an individual context. In other words, it will present the reality that for type-two diabetes, in particular, the necessary changes that will treat and control glucose levels form part of the overall requirements for eating well, being healthy and living life to the full. As such they should be carried out irrespective of a diagnosis and should be seen as a mechanism to stop the occurrence of the condition in the first place. In short for type-two diabetes, prevention is absolutely possible and is most certainly preferable to cure. This book will explain all of these points in very strong and hopefully engaging terms.

Finally, during the course of the text, you will read of various studies and research findings. This research forms the bedrock of the central assertion of the text, which is simply that eating a balanced diet and performing some form of exercise on a daily basis, will definitely help prevent Type-two diabetes. I have endeavoured to find research that is as much as possible written in lay terms. The reader is actively encouraged to follow up on this *"primary scientific literature"* and delve in and follow up in any direction they see fit. In a similar vein, it is impossible to present a detailed history of a condition such as diabetes in and so the reader is encouraged to view the hyperlinks contained in the writing as a helpful series of well-lit sign posts.

As with many scientific terms, diabetes is derived from the language of Greece which is, of course, Greek! Approximately 1800 years ago a physician (a doctor to you and I) called Aretus the Cappadocian first coined the term *"diabainein"*. He wrote of patients who were frequently urinating (polyuria), which is a key symptom of what is now term diabetes. However, knowledge of the condition can be traced back to ancient China, where physicians noticed that the urine of some people was more attractive to insects because it was sweeter; we now know this is due to elevated levels of glucose.

In the China of thousands of years ago diabetes was called *"sweet urine disease"*, hmmm Nice! Without any intent to amuse the word diabetes actually means syphon in the Greek language. In 1675 a British scientist named Thomas Willis added the word Mellitus to the Medieval Latin word diabetes. In Latin *"mel"* translates to honey, hence we can bring all of these strands together and state that diabetes mellitus is loosely translated as a condition in which sweet water is siphoned. All of this is to impact that human beings have been aware of diabetes for several thousand years. What is perhaps less understood is the fact that diabetes is largely preventable and it causes a whole range of life-threatening conditions which kill millions people all over the world every year.

According to the UK National Health Service (NHS), the total number of people over 16 who had either type one (T1) or type-two (T2) diabetes in 2010 was approximately 3 million people. This figure doubles up on the number recorded in 1996, at least if the figures from a UK charity are to be believed. In any writing concerning a medical condition authority (or ethos) is absolutely essential. Charities, NGO's and their ilk work exceptionally hard on getting the numbers "right" and making sure that the science and statistics behind producing them are equally stringent. After all, they are spending supporter cash on developing research! Thus, if you happen to be experiencing diabetes at the sharp end, then you will be pleased to know that research findings produced by organisations such as www.diabetes.org.uk are pretty much hammering the proverbial nail on the head. With this in mind, the numbers involved in the UK alone are truly staggering. For instance, diabetes UK estimates that by 2030 the number of individuals experiencing diabetes or a medical complication caused by it will exceed 4.5 million people, by 2035 the figure could exceed 6 million. Overall, the ratio of T2 to T1 diabetes is 9:1, meaning that 90% of all cases of diabetes are of the preventable or curable variety. This notion will be demonstrated empirically below.

In addition, approximately 1 million people in the UK are thought to have "diabetes" but have yet to be diagnosed. The number of people across the UK (and the wider world) who are considered to be pre-diabetic is very difficult to quantify, but it is believed to number in the tens of millions. A person is considered pre-diabetic if their blood sugar (glucose) level is outside of the normal homeostatic range, but they have yet to develop the symptoms of T2 diabetes.

The focus of the condition centres on the blood concentration of a wholly nondescript molecule known as glucose ($C_6H_{12}O_6$) and its interaction with the hormone insulin. This relationship will be explored in some detail below.

Glucose is the simplest carbohydrate (a substance which is composed only of atoms of hydrogen, carbon, and oxygen) and is in a very real sense the *"fuel"* which drives our metabolism. The compound is water soluble and so can be transported throughout the body to all of our cells. In living cells glucose is chemically converted to carbon dioxide and water thus providing the necessary energy to drive the biochemical reactions (metabolism) which keep us alive. Glucose is particularly important for the human brain; the organ constitutes some 3% of our overall body weight (well mass to be pedantic) but consumes some 20-25% of the glucose in the blood in the process of respiration. Put simply, if the blood sugar (glucose) level remains *"too high"* for *"too long"* the probability of developing full diabetes will increase. An important caveat exists and it concerns diabetes in children, in this frame we are talking about any person less than 16 years old. Approximately 25,000 children in the UK have diabetes; however, over 97% of this is T1 diabetes with the majority of the difference being made up of T2 diabetes. This fact should present a glaringly obvious question to the reader which is **"why does the trend reverse in adulthood?"**

The incidence of T2 diabetes can be directly correlated with the incidence of obesity and so it is fair to say that T2 diabetes is very much a disease of the affluent world. Well, to be more precise it is a disease correlated with the eating what is known in as the western diet. This is reflected in research from organisations such as the World Health Organisation (WHO). A recent fact sheet asserts that *"a diabetes epidemic is underway"*. If you think this is alarmist or sensationalist statement then you need to keep reading. In 1985 approximately 30 million people around the world were diagnosed with T1 or T2 diabetes, once again roughly 90% were found in the latter category. Within ten years the number had rocketed to approximately 140 million, by the turn of the 20th century some 180 million people were recorded as being diabetic. The upward trend looks set to continue such that by 2025 the WHO estimates that a minimum of 300 million people will have developed diabetes. Make no mistake about it diabetes is a serious health condition which if left treated will adversely affect the symptoms which keep a person alive. It will if not adequately treated result in premature death or profound physical disability. Currently, approximately 4 million people die annually due to complications caused by diabetes; this figure translates to roughly 9% of the global death rate. The vast majority of these recorded deaths are down to diseases of the heart and blood vessels (cardiovascular) and occur prematurely whilst the person is for want of a better phrase *"in their prime"*. In addition, if left untreated diabetes can lead to stroke, diseases of the nervous system, blindness, and renal failure as well as other undesirable and life-threatening conditions.

According to the International Diabetes Foundation (IDF), a global diabetes charity, as of 2013 over 387 million people have diabetes. The future prognosis from this organisation is comparable to that of the WHO, as the IDF predict that some 600 million people will have diabetes within 2-3 decades.

Overall, it is estimated that about $376 Billion was spent globally in 2010 on both treating diabetes and complications arising from its incidence. This huge number represents approximately 10% of the total health expenditure. It is estimated that by 2030 if the situation does not improve then we are looking at an expenditure of $490 billion dollars. Yet the real tragedy is that approximately 90% of all deaths from diabetes are preventable and increasingly it is the less affluent countries that are bearing the brunt of diabetes care. To put it in purely financial terms 90% of the 376 billion dollar figure could have been spent elsewhere. I wonder how much good work the NGO's of the world could do with such financial clout. For the UK, the figures make equally grim reading, as of 2012 the UK spent £14 billion on treating diabetes and related conditions. The breakdown matches the ratio outlined above because an incredible 87% of the UK figure was spent treating the consequences of T2 diabetes. The NHS, in particular, would surely benefit from an additional £11.718 billion per year every year, without actually having to carry out ludicrous actions, such as shutting Accident and Emergency facilities across the country (the UK). None of this is to partition blame and lay the ills of the world at the door of people who have acquired T2 diabetes, (speaking personally I have no take with such arguments) but is to make a point. If a condition is so preventable, the obvious question is to ask *"why does this bizarre situation exist in the first place?"* The simple answer is that most diabetes is acquired and not inherited. The next section will explain why this is so.

Maintaining an optimal level of glucose (blood sugar) in the circulatory system (bloodstream) is an example of homoeostasis. It means keeping the internal environment the same so that all biological processes can occur as they should irrespective of external conditions. The term homoeostasis was first coined by a French scientist called Claude Bernard in 1865. Although we shall be looking almost exclusively at blood sugar levels, the reader must realise that the human organism strives to keep all variables within homeostatic limits no matter the activities of the organism. In terms of the metabolism of glucose, the actions of two hormones insulin and glucagon facilitate the maintenance of the correct glucose level in the bloodstream. The hormones act such that the body stores chemical energy in the form of glycogen and fats in times of plenty. If the pantry (so to speak) becomes dry during the dietary change, exercise or in any time of survival crises then the same hormones act to ensure that chemical energy in the form of glucose is released into the general circulation providing the energy the body needs. Clearly, the optimal blood sugar level will vary between individual people and is subject to many variables. Hence there is no definite upper or lower limit of acceptable glucose concentration in the blood. The average person can expect their glucose level to be recorded as between 4 and 10 mmol/l (mili-moles per litre). The designation is the accepted global counting unit and is a standard mechanism by which to measure glucose concentrations in the blood stream. The above figure general refers to a situation in which the person has not eaten for approximately 8 hours.

When a person absorbs glucose into their blood stream, for example as a result of eating a carbohydrate rich meal the baseline level can increase by as much as 25 to 35%. The increase in concentration is picked up by the hypothalamus (part of the brain which regulates the release of hormones) which stimulates the pancreas to release insulin. The result is the conversion of glucose into glycogen (glycogenesis). Insulin also increases the rate of cellular respiration, which is the conversion of glucose to water and carbon dioxide.

Glycogenesis is most effective in the liver, muscles, and adipose (fat) cells. All things being equal glycogenesis returns the blood glucose concentration to within homeostatic limits. Once homoeostasis has been achieved, the secretion of insulin stops and any excess insulin is excreted via the renal (kidney) system. Very roughly a healthy adult human being will store about 100g of glycogen in the liver and this is an immediate source of energy should blood sugar levels drop toward the lower limit. When blood sugar levels drop toward the lower homeostatic limit, the hypothalamus stimulates the pancreas to release the hormone glucagon, which has the opposite effect to insulin. In other words, glycogen is converted to glucose (gluconeogenesis) and the rate of cellular respiration decreases. Gluconeogenesis functions by increasing blood sugar levels and glycogenesis functions by decreasing blood sugar levels and the hormones operate antagonistically. In other words maintaining an optimal glucose concentration is a constant see-saw process and perfectly normal aspect of healthy metabolism. The reader should not view the presence of either hormone as an *"either or"* scenario, there is always glucagon and insulin circulating in the bloodstream. As with our diet, the body is attempting to maintain homoeostasis and to achieve this both hormones must be present.

Should glucose levels fall below the minimum homoeostatic limit and not be replaced (hypoglycaemia) then all respiring cells begin to lose their primary source of energy. The symptoms of hyperglycemia (insulin shock) are generally shaking, palpitations, severe hunger pangs, and very rapid heartbeat. This set of symptoms is caused by the stress hormone epinephrine (adrenaline), which is secreted by the adrenal glands in response to the low sugar concentration. If the concentration of glucose cannot be increased then brain cells will eventually seize up resulting in unconsciousness coma and then death. The opposite scenario (hyperglycemia) occurs where the body cannot remove glucose from the body even when levels of glycogen drop to their absolute minimum levels (such as after eating). The body cannot metabolise enough glucose and the condition we know as diabetes (Diabetes Mellitus DM) presents itself. In other words, hyperglycemia is the condition which causes both T1 and T2 DM. Both forms of diabetes produce a whole set of symptoms which mean that the body is not properly regulating its blood glucose levels. It may helpful to view hyperglycemia as a form of glucose poisoning and the symptoms of diabetes are a consequence of the body attempting to detoxify itself. Overall, either the pancreas does not produce enough (if any) insulin or the insulin produced is ineffective. So, what's the difference between T1 and T2 diabetes?

 In T1 diabetes the specialist cells which produce insulin have been destroyed by the immune system and so no matter how high the level of glucose in the body, insulin is not produced. Hence the homeostatic process outlined above breaks down. As will be outlined in chapter three a person with T1 diabetes requires a lifetime of treatment to maintain the correct levels of insulin in the blood stream. Hence T1 diabetes is often referred to as *"insulin-dependent or juvenile onset"* diabetes. In general terms, T1 diabetes expresses itself during adolescence, but it can arise in middle age. Researchers in the field believe that a genetic basis for the condition exists but it is widely believed to be caused by an autoimmune response. Put simply an auto-immune response occurs when the immune system attacks the cells of the body. This happens because the immune system (B and T cells) "see" the healthy cells as a pathogen and act accordingly. There are approximately 100 autoimmune diseases, ranging from Irritable Bowel Syndrome (IBS), Chrons disease and Psoriasis to Arthritis as well as MS, in short, there are some right nasties under the moniker of autoimmune disease!

The response can be triggered by foreign micro-organisms (pathogenic or not), prescribed drugs which *"confuse"* the immune response. As yet science cannot tell us the exact mechanisms which cause these diseases but researchers believe that a genetic basis exists which makes a person more susceptible than others. Hence, in very general terms T1 diabetes can be viewed as an inherited condition (although this is not strictly speaking true). However, researchers prefer to view T1 diabetes as autoimmune diseases and not an inherited genetic disorder. In the case of T1 diabetes, the *"confused"* immune system destroys the *"islet of Langerhans cells"* which is a specialist structure located in the pancreas. A healthy pancreas contains up to 3 million of these insulin-making cells which are approximately 1/50th of the total number of cells in the pancreas itself. One area of research into T1 diabetes concerns the action of a family of viruses known as Coxsackie B Enteroviruses (CBE). These viruses have an incubation period ranging from 2 to 6 days and are the cause of diseases such as foot and mouth and meningitis. The CBE virus family has been implicated as a cause of T1DM but the mechanism is far from understood. The main focus of this Book is on the intertwined roles of diet and lifestyle choices on acquiring T2 diabetes. However, if the reader wishes to explore the genetic and environmental basis of type 1 diabetes then this link is an excellent starting position: http://bit.ly/diapedia.

T2 DM is an entirely different ball game as it is linked to a wholly undesirable confluence of obesity, bad diet and a lack of exercise and occurs generally in individuals aged over 40 years old. Having said that the incidence of T2 diabetes in children under 16 is steadily increasing and the reasons are essentially the same as for adults. In terms of genetics and hereditary T2, diabetes would be classified as an *"acquired characteristic"* and that means it can be treated, but it is obviously better to think in terms of prevention. In T2 (non-insulin-dependent or adult onset) DM the person experiences broadly similar symptoms to those caused by T1 diabetes. However, because of the chronic and less severe nature as well as the wide range of possible symptoms T2 DM can be difficult to diagnose. Therefore, a person may be well on the way to developing the serious complications mentioned previously in this chapter, but may not know it. In other words, they are prediabetic. Hence we have another crystal clear argument for following the dietary advice intertwined throughout this series of books. To underpin the importance of prevention T2 diabetes is beginning to make its presence felt in children who are overweight or obese (because the diet is unbalanced) and do not exercise. For example, in the year 2000, the first confirmed cases of T2 diabetes were confirmed in Pakistani, Indian and Arabian girls aged 9 to 16. Furthermore, new Research from the US demonstrates that over 90% of all children that are overweight or obese have developed T2 diabetes. These figures themselves are occurring in a population where a third of all children fall into the overweight/obese category. The next chapter will seek to outline the role of diet in precipitating this wholly preventable epidemic.

Do you want to carry on reading?

If so, visit www.amazon.com or www.viddapublishing.com to purchase your full copy of "DIABETES: PREVENTION & REVERSAL with a SIRTFOOD & PLANT-BASED DIET" by John Hodges & Ted Gif.

Other Books by VIDDA Publishing

THE MEDICINE ON YOUR PLATE Series

Understanding Disease, Prevention & The Importance of Plant Based Nutrition and Diet

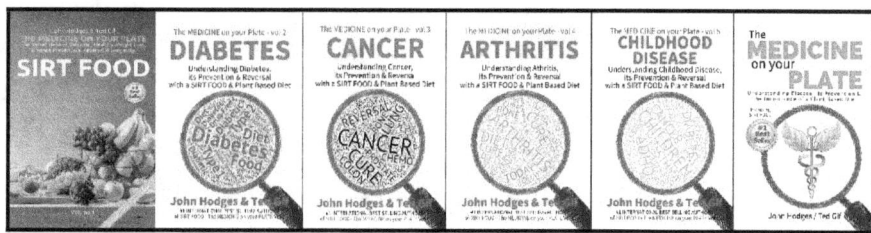

GREEN UP YOUR LIFE Series (Also in Spanish & Bilingual)

Take control of your health and wellbeing by introducing Natural, Eco-Friendly habits into your daily routine.

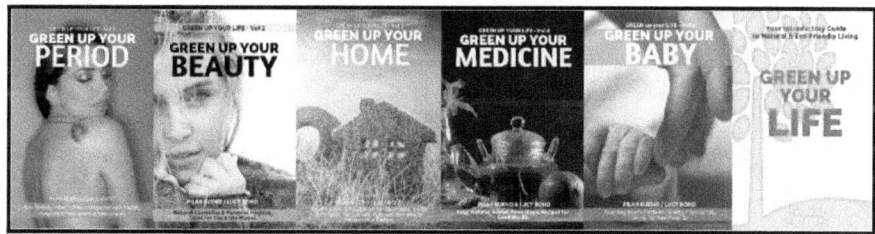

DOG TALES Series

Stories of Loyalty, Heroism & Devotion

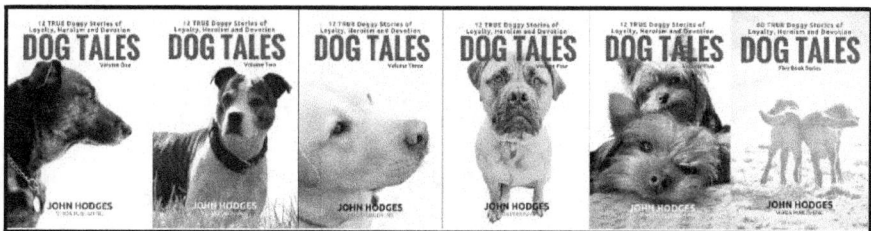

BUSINESS, INCOME & SOCIAL MEDIA Series
How to Promote, Market & Create Business with Social Media

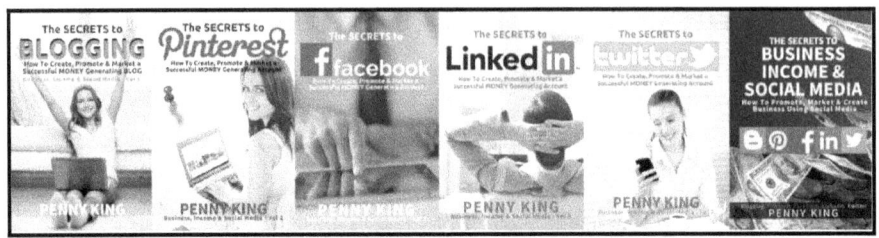

MINDFULNESS: MAKE A RESOLUTION TO BE HAPPY (Available in Spanish & Bilingual)
Make yourself smile every day and banish stress and anxiety

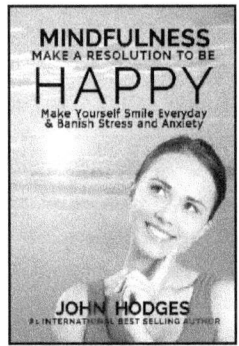

INTRODUCING GENETICALLY MODIFIED ORGANISMS - GMO
The History, Research and The TRUTH You're Not Being Told

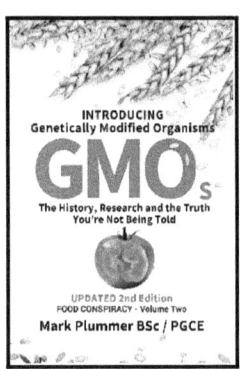

FOOD CONSPIRACY: WHAT HAPPENED TO OUR BREAD?
The Chorleywood Bread Process

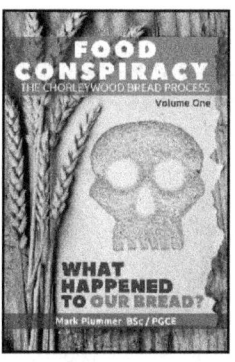

NATURAL WILD WINES
A Guide To Making Delicious Home Made Wine. Tips, Equipment, Recipes & Foraging Wild Fruits, Flowers & Herbs

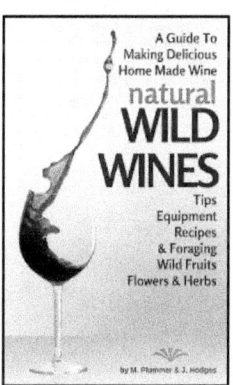

www.viddapublishing.com/books.html

Connect with John Hodges

If this book has helped you in any way or inspired you to take control of your own health and nutrition, it makes me a very happy man.

You can check out my publishing blog "Living Like You Mean It" (**viddapublishing.blogspot.co.uk**) for helpful tips, inspiration and updates on new books and free promotions coming soon.

You can also follow me on:

Twitter: twitter.com/VIDDAPublishing

John Hodges' Facebook: www.facebook.com/people/John-Hodges/550153788

VIDDA Publishing's Facebook: www.facebook.com/viddapublishing

For your Healthy, Nutritious, Green and Cruelty Free products, equipment and gadgets, visit our online **VIDDA Health Stores** (US: **bit.ly/VIDDAstore** & UK: **bit.ly/VIDDAstoreUK**).

Also, for our favourite supplier of nutrients, sprouting seeds and health products, visit **bit.ly/BuyWholeFoodsOnline**

If you have any questions at all, please feel free to contact me at: **viddapublishing.com/contact.html**

Wishing you the best of Health.

John Hodges

www.viddapublishing.com

www.themedicineonyourplate.com

www.sirtfood.com

www.greenupyourlife.org

www.ecologizatuvida.com

Glossary of terms

Alveoli - any of the many tiny air sacs of the lungs which allow for rapid gaseous exchange.

Autophagy - is a normal physiological process in the body that deals with the destruction of cells in the body. It maintains homeostasis or normal functioning by protein degradation and turnover of the destroyed cell organelles for new cell formation.

Carbonic Anhydrase - The **carbonic anhydrases** (or carbonate dehydratases) form a family of enzymes that **catalyze** the rapid interconversion of **carbon** dioxide and water to bicarbonate and protons (or vice versa), a reversible reaction that occurs relatively slowly in the absence of a catalyst.

CJD - **Creutzfeldt-Jakob disease** (CJD) is a rare, degenerative, invariably fatal brain disorder. [1] Although the agent of sporadic **CJD** (sCJD), the most common type of **CJD**, differs from the agent of bovine spongiform encephalopathy (BSE) or "mad cow disease", sCJD is often confused with the human form of BSE.

Cytoplasm - the material or protoplasm within a living cell, excluding the nucleus.

Cytosol - the aqueous component of the cytoplasm of a cell, within which various organelles and particles are suspended.

Enzymes - a substance produced by a living organism which acts as a catalyst to bring about a specific biochemical reaction.

Golgi - an organelle in eukaryotic cells that stores and modifies proteins for specific functions and prepares them for transport to other parts of the cell. The **Golgi** apparatus is usually near the cell nucleus and consists of a stack of flattened sacs

Homeostasis - the tendency towards a relatively stable equilibrium between interdependent elements, especially as maintained by physiological processes.

Homeostatically - The tendency of the body to seek and maintain a condition of balance or equilibrium within its internal environment, even when faced with external changes. A simple example of homeostasis is the body's ability to maintain an internal temperature around 98.6 degrees Fahrenheit, whatever the temperature outside.

Metabolites - a substance formed in or necessary for metabolism.

Mitosis - a type of cell division that results in two daughter cells each having the same number and kind of chromosomes as the parent nucleus, typical of ordinary tissue growth.

Organelles - any of a number of organized or specialized structures within a living cell.

Polyphenol - a compound containing more than one phenolic hydroxyl group.

Ribosomes - a minute particle consisting of RNA and associated proteins found in large numbers in the cytoplasm of living cells. They bind to messenger RNA and transfer RNA to synthesize polypeptides and proteins.

U.N.E.S.C.O. - United Nations Educational, Scientific, and Cultural Organization.

W.H.O. – World Health Organisation

Useful Websites

http://nutritionfacts.org

http://www.naturalnews.com

http://nutritiondata.self.com

https://www.pinterest.com/coco942001/save-yourself/

https://www.pinterest.com/coco942001/clean-food-recipes/

https://viddapublishing.com

http://viddapublishing.blogspot.co.uk/

Sources

http://www.sciencedirect.com/science/article/pii/S00062952
11005697

http://www.nejm.org/doi/full/10.1056/NEJMoa1200303

http://www.theguardian.com/science/blog/2014/apr/11/resv
eratrol-wonder-chemical-red-wine-cancer-ageing

http://www.xconomy.com/boston/2013/03/12/glaxosmithkli
ne-shuts-down-sirtris-five-years-after-720m-buyout/

http://www.nature.com/neuro/journal/v1/n1/pdf/nn0598_6
9.pdf

http://www.theguardian.com/society/2014/nov/20/obesity-
bigger-cost-than-war-and-terror

http://www.cancer.gov/about-cancer/causes-
prevention/risk/diet/tea-fact-sheet

http://www.mdpi.com/1420-3049/12/5/946

http://www.nature.com/news/sirtuin-protein-linked-to-
longevity-in-mammals-1.10074

http://ajcn.nutrition.org/content/81/2/341.full.pdf+html

http://www.rsc.org/chemistryworld/2013/06/resveratrol-
red-wine-heart-disease-podcast

http://mcb.asm.org/content/23/9/3173.full.pdf+html

http://jnci.oxfordjournals.org/content/89/24/1881.full.pdf+h
tml

http://cshperspectives.cshlp.org/content/4/12/a013102.full.pdf+html

http://www.sciencedirect.com/science/article/pii/S092544391
3001804

http://www.sciencedirect.com/science/article/pii/S000989811
2005773

http://sciencelife.uchospitals.edu/2014/10/16/two-faced-gene-sirt6-prevents-some-cancers-but-promotes-sun-induced-skin-cancer/

http://www.the-scientist.com/?articles.view/articleNo/13625/title/Mapping-Subtelomeres/

http://www.ncbi.nlm.nih.gov/pubmed/18607383

http://www.kurzweilai.net/why-sirt1-in-your-brain-may-keep-you-smart

http://www.ncbi.nlm.nih.gov/pmc/articles/PMC3249911/

http://www.ncbi.nlm.nih.gov/pmc/articles/PMC2727669/

http://www.ncbi.nlm.nih.gov/pmc/articles/PMC3117983/

http://www.chem.ucla.edu/harding/ec_tutorials/tutorial43.pdf

http://www.ncbi.nlm.nih.gov/pmc/articles/PMC2835915/

http://www.nature.com/ncomms/2014/140401/ncomms4557/full/ncomms4557.html

http://www.ncbi.nlm.nih.gov/pmc/articles/PMC2020845/#R 10

http://www.ncbi.nlm.nih.gov/pmc/articles/PMC2020845/

http://www.sciencedaily.com/releases/2013/03/13032713334 1.html

http://www.theatlantic.com/health/archive/2014/03/science-compared-every-diet-and-the-winner-is-real-food/284595/

http://www.theguardian.com/lifeandstyle/2013/jun/19/japan ese-diet-live-to-100

https://elainehastings.wordpress.com/tag/mediterranean-diet/

http://www.hindawi.com/journals/omcl/2013/707421/

http://genesdev.cshlp.org/content/27/19/2072.full.pdf+html

http://www.nature.com/cddis/journal/v1/n1/pdf/cddis20091 7a.pdf

http://www.nature.com/cddis/journal/v1/n1/pdf/cddis20098 a.pdf

http://jn.nutrition.org/content/10/1/63.short

Books and further reading

Not on the label Felicity Lawrence, Penguin books 2004.

http://www.mckinsey.com/insights/economic_studies/how_the_world_could_better_fight_obesity

http://www.foodforlife.org.uk/what-is-food-for-life

http://www.nationalobesityforum.org.uk/media/PDFs/StateOfTheNationsWaistlineObesityintheUKAnalysisandExpectations.pdf

http://www.sciencedaily.com/search/?keyword=sirtuins+%2Bcalorie+restriction#gsc.tab=0&gsc.q=sirtuins%20%2Bcalorie%20restriction&gsc.page=1

www.ingramcontent.com/pod-product-compliance
Lightning Source LLC
Chambersburg PA
CBHW051647170526
45167CB00001B/365